In Clinical Practice

Taking a practical approach to clinical medicine, this series of smaller reference books is designed for the trainee physician, primary care physician, nurse practitioner and other general medical professionals to understand each topic covered. The coverage is comprehensive but concise and is designed to act as a primary reference tool for subjects across the field of medicine.

More information about this series at http://www.springer.com/series/13483

Dmitriy Kireyev • Judy Hung
Editors

Cardiac Imaging
in Clinical Practice

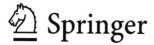 Springer

Editors
Dmitriy Kireyev
Division of Cardiology
Massachusetts General Hospital
Boston
Massachusetts
USA

Judy Hung
Division of Cardiology
Massachusetts General Hospital
Boston
Massachusetts
USA

ISSN 2199-6652   ISSN 2199-6660   (electronic)
In Clinical Practice
ISBN 978-3-319-21457-3   ISBN 978-3-319-21458-0   (eBook)
DOI 10.1007/978-3-319-21458-0

Library of Congress Control Number: 2015954723

Springer Cham Heidelberg New York Dordrecht London

Springer International Publishing AG Switzerland is part of Springer Science+Business Media (www.springer.com)

Contents

Contributors

Sanjeev A. Francis, MD Cardio-Oncology Program, Cardiac MRI/CT Program, Massachusetts General Hospital, Boston, MA, USA

Brain Ghoshhajra, MD Department of Radiology, Massachusetts General Hospital, Boston, MA, USA

Lanqi Hua, BS, RDCS, FASE Cardiac Ultrasound Laboratory, Massachusetts General Hospital, Boston, MA, USA

Judy Hung, MD Echocardiography, Division of Cardiology, Massachusetts General Hospital, Boston, MA, USA

Asaad A. Khan, MBBS, MRCP Division of Cardiology, Massachusetts General Hospital, Harvard Medical School, Boston, MA, USA

Dmitriy Kireyev, MD Echocardiography, Division of Cardiology, Massachusetts General Hospital, Boston, MA, USA

Marcello Panagia, MD, PhD Cardiology Division, Massachusetts General Hospital, Boston, MA, USA

Jonathan Scheske, MD Department of Radiology, Massachusetts General Hospital, Boston, MA, USA

Parmanand Singh, MD Division of Cardiology, Department of Radiology, Weill Cornell Medical College, New York Presbyterian Hospital, New York, NY, USA

Michael F. Wilson, MD Nuclear Cardiology and Cardiovascular CT Angiography, State University of New York at Buffalo, Kaleida Health Hospitals, Buffalo, NY, USA

Chapter 1
Basics of Ultrasound Physics

Dmitriy Kireyev and Judy Hung

Ultrasound – Refers to sound waves with frequencies higher than 20 kHz, which is higher than the frequencies perceptible to the human ear.

Ultrasound waves travel at a speed of approximately 1540 m/s in soft tissue such as muscle.

- Sound of different frequencies travels through the same media at same speed.
- High frequency sound has lower penetration.
- The higher the frequency, the smaller the object that reflects sound without scattering.
- $C = \lambda \upsilon$, where c – speed of sound λ – wavelength, υ – frequency
- Speed in media is proportional to density and elasticity (which is proportional to temperature). Thus sound travels faster in soft tissue than air and faster in metal than soft tissue.
- Ultrasound waves can reflect and refract when they are interacting borders between different media (Fig. 1.1)

D. Kireyev, MD (✉) • J. Hung, MD
Echocardiography, Division of Cardiology,
Massachusetts General Hospital, Boston, MA, USA
e-mail: dimonk5@yahoo.com;
JHUNG@mgh.harvard.edu

D. Kireyev, J. Hung (eds.), *Cardiac Imaging in Clinical Practice*, In Clinical Practice,
DOI 10.1007/978-3-319-21458-0_1,
© Springer International Publishing Switzerland 2016

1

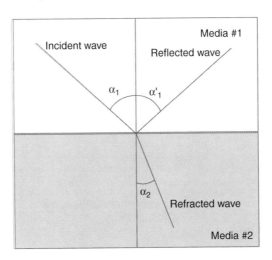

FIGURE 1.1 Ultrasound waves both reflect and refract when they come to border between two media with different physical properties

Transducer can be focused only in near field

$L_n = r^2 / \lambda = r^2 \upsilon / c$, Where L_n – length of near field, λ – wavelength, υ – frequency, r – radius of the transducer, c- speed of sound in media

$\text{Sin } \alpha = 0.61 / r$ – divergence of beam in the far field

Snell's law: calculates angle of refraction

$\text{Sin} \alpha_1 / \text{Sin} \alpha_2 = V_1 / V_2 = n_2 / n_1$ where n is index of refraction

Spatial Resolution: refers to the smallest distance in which 2 points can be distinguished as separate. There are two types of spatial resolution; axial and lateral (Fig. 1.2).

Axial resolution: refers to ability to resolve 2 points in the direction of the ultrasound beam (axial direction or depth); proportional to λ, υ, and duration of transmitted pulse. Typical axial resolution for cardiac ultrasound is

Lateral resolution: refers to ability to resolve 2 points in a perpendicular plane from the ultrasound beam (along the sides of the beam); proportional to beam width

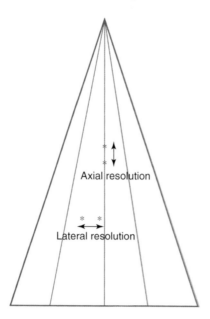

FIGURE 1.2 Definition of axial and lateral resolution

Temporal Resolution: refers to ability to resolve 2 points that has moved over time; is quantified as the frame rate; frame rates can be improved by narrowing imaging sector, decreasing depth, and decreasing line density

Absorption: refers to when sound amplitude is weakened due to inner friction (viscosity)

– Energy transferred to heat
– Scattering occurs at all the interfaces

Attenuation refers to decrease in sound amplitude from reflection of sound wave

– Attenuation increases as frequency of sound wave increases (can reflect off smaller interfaces)

Half value level – distance sound travels before intensity goes to 50 %

In tissue attenuation is 1 dB/cm/MHz

Transducer

Transducers contain piezoelectric elements which are made of metallic crystals that can transfer sound waves to electric signals and vice versa. These physical elements are responsible for the mechanoelectric transduction of ultrasound to electric data.

Diagram Basic Elements in an Ultrasound Probe (Fig. 1.3)

1. Piezoelectric element. It is responsible for generating pulses and receiving the ultrasound signals
2. Marching layers. Due to significant impedance differences between the transducer and the human body a significant amount of reflection can occur at the interface between the two (this is also a reason why we use gel to eliminate the air between the probe and the body). These layers increase

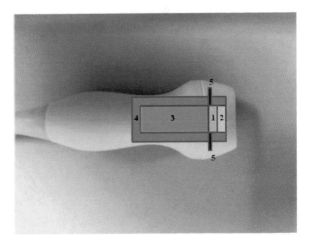

FIGURE 1.3 Diagram of basic components in ultrasound transducer. Please review text for more details

the acoustic power, sensitivity and axial resolution. The thickness of each layer is ¼ of transducer basic frequency to minimize internal reverberations within the probe.

3. Dampening material. It dampens the vibration of the piezoelectric element allowing to limit output time (thus improving range resolution) and absorbing the waves released from the back end of the transducer

4. Shielding material which limits the effect of outside vibrations on a piezoelectric element

5. Electrical connections – they both provide initial energy to excite the piezoelectric element and transmit back to the machine the electric signal which is generated by the piezoelectric element upon encountering reflected ultrasound waves

Transducer Frequency

- Determined by thickness of piezoelectric element
- Shock-excitation of a piezoelectric crystal results in transmission of sound energy from both front and back faces of crystal
- When thickness of element is ½ λ, the reflected and transmitted stresses at each surface reinforce each other and transducer resonates at maximum displacement amplitude –this is referred to as fundamental resonant frequency of the transducer
- when thickness is λ, the stresses at each surface are opposite – then displacement amplitude is minimal
- the thickness of piezoelectric element is inversely proportional to frequency generated (thickness proportional to λ proportional to c/υ)

Transducer Damping

- Piezoelectric elements used in transducers have long response to excitation – long ultrasound pulse

- Damping material is placed behind transducer to decrease length of ringing. This material also absorbs sound energy emitted from the back of the transducer
- High degree of damping decreases both pulse duration and sensitivity
- Impedance matching layers:
  - acoustic impedance of transducer is 25 times higher than that of human body.
  - acoustic impedance difference can cause 96 % reflective loss at transducer-skin interface.
  - Impedance matching layers increase power input, sensitivity, bandwidth and axial resolution.

Transducer Frequency

- Increases in frequency improve resolution but also decrease penetration into structures.
- Typical transducer frequencies are 2.0–2.5 mHz (in adults), 3.5 MHz (in children), and 5–12 MHz (in neonates and young children).

Doppler Basics

Doppler effect is a change of frequency of sound for an observer as his or her position changes relative to the source. (Do you remember how the sound of fire truck changes when it comes first towards you and then drives away?)

$$\upsilon = \upsilon \text{ initial} \left(\frac{c + V \; receiver}{c + V \; transducer} \right)$$

Where υ is frequency, c is the speed of sound in particular media and V is velocity

The ultrasound transducer emits an ultrasound wave which upon reaching target is reflected back to transducer. The change in frequency allows the machine to determine the speed of moving object.

An Extremely Simplified Explanation of How Ultrasound Waves Define Structures

Ultrasound waves are sent by the probe, reflected by an object and these reflected waves are also received by the transducer. The package which returns to the probe includes a combination of reflected and deflected waves from multiple surfaces created by interface between tissues with different impedances. Piezoelectric crystal converts the waves into oscillating electrical signals (ES). ES has several components that may be analyzed: the amplitude, the phase and the duration of pulse train. If one now imagines an oscillator which sweeps the signal up and down on the screen which is used to produce an image, the reconstructed image will represent a single line which is a vertical representation of "cut-through" image showing points where change in density of tissue which ultrasound penetrates occurs. If you imagine a screen divided in x-y plane of standard Cartesian coordinate system, the Y axis can be controlled by the timing of the oscillator while if one makes the brightness of the dots on the screen proportional which is proportional to the reflection point. Thus you get a line which is similar to producing an infinitely thin slice of the heart and then getting a vertical view of it. This is the basis of the B-mode echocardiography. However, imagine that you can move this line along the X-axis at certain speed – the curves created by the dots will represent the above mentioned infinitely small slice of the heart moving with time (hence the term "M-mode"). To take it to another level: make the probe oscillate the initial ultrasound signal and reconstruct it properly on the screen as the side view of multiple very thin slices of the heart (similar to creating a combination of multiple B-mode lines on one screen with the relative location of lines corresponding to the locations of the cut planes through the heart). Now, create an image on the screen, completely erase it and create another one fraction of a second later. By repeating this process with extremely high speed one can show the movement of a heart plane which may show movement of multiple structures. In a way it is similar to the initial stages of cinematography. The first motion picture was created by E J Muybridge in 1878. He essentially took pictures of a horse at a trot (taken by multiple cameras along the track). Then he put the images as silhouettes on a rotating glass disk (in the correct sequence). Fast motion of this disk created an impression of a movie (if you are interested, the device was called zoopraxiscope).

Chapter 2
Views and Structures

Lanqi Hua and Dmitriy Kireyev

Standard imaging views used in transthoracic echocardiography are obtained from parasternal, apical, subcostal and suprasternal windows. Figure 2.1 shows the imaging planes of these views as they relate to the cardiac structures.

Transducer positions and related echocardiographic images for parasternal long axis views are shown in Fig. 2.2.

Transducer positions and related echocardiographic images for parasternal short axis views are shown in Fig. 2.3.

Transducer positions and related echocardiographic images for apical views are shown in Fig. 2.4.

Transducer positions and related echocardiographic images for subcostal views are shown in Fig. 2.5

Transducer positions and related echocardiographic images for suprasternal are shown in Fig. 2.6.

Transducer positions and related echocardiographic images for right parasternal long axis views are shown in Fig. 2.7.

L. Hua, BS, RDCS, FASE
Cardiac Ultrasound Laboratory,
Massachusetts General Hospital, Boston, MA, USA

D. Kireyev, MD (✉)
Echocardiography, Division of Cardiology,
Massachusetts General Hospital, Boston, MA, USA
e-mail: dimonk5@yahoo.com

D. Kireyev, J. Hung (eds.), *Cardiac Imaging in Clinical Practice*, In Clinical Practice,
DOI 10.1007/978-3-319-21458-0_2,
© Springer International Publishing Switzerland 2016

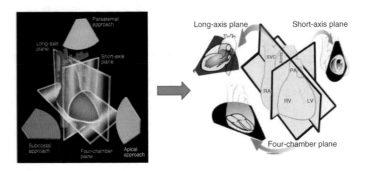

FIGURE 2.1 Image of the heart showing the right parsternal, parasternal, apical and subcostal windows as they relate to the cardiac structures

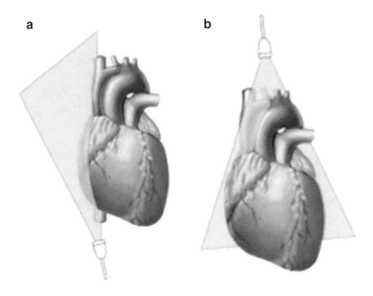

FIGURE 2.2 Image of the heart showing the suprasternal (**b**) and subcostal (**a**) windows as they relate to the cardiac structures

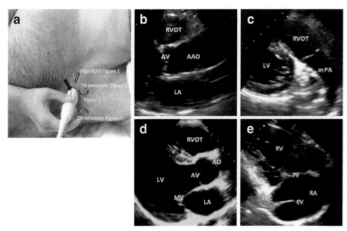

Parasternal long-axis view

FIGURE 2.3 Transducer positions and echocardiographic images for parasternal long axis views. (**a**) Probe position. (**b**) Ascending aorta view. (**c**) RV outflow view. (**d**) Parasternal long-axis view. (**e**) RV inflow view. *Abbreviations*: *LA* left atrium, *RCC* and *NCC* right coronary and non-coronary cusps of aortic valve, *AAO* ascending Aorta, *RVOT* right ventricular outflow tract, *LV* left ventricle, *mPA* main pulmonary artery, *AMVL* and *PMVL* anterior and posterior mitral valve leaflets, *ATVL* and *PTVL* anterior and posterior mitral valve leaflets, *RA* right atrium, *CS* coronary sinus, *IVC* inferior vena cava, *EV* Eustachian valve

Coronary sinus can be viewed in the parasternal long axis window and also a modified apical four chamber view in which the transducer is tilted posteriorly (Fig. 2.8).

Although the left atrial appendage is best imaged using transesophageal echocardiography, it can sometimes be viewed well by transthoracic imaging (Fig. 2.9).

The proximal portions of the coronary arteries as seen in a parasternal short axis view (Figs. 2.10 and 2.11).

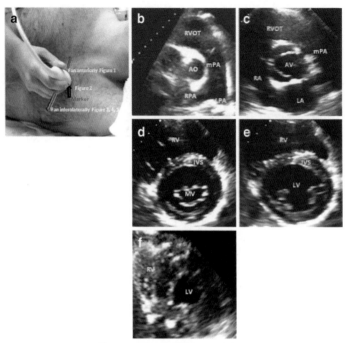

Parasternal short-axis view

FIGURE 2.4 Transducer positions and images for parasternal short axis views. (**a**) Probe position. (**b**) Pulmonary bifurcation view. (**c**) AV level. (**d**) MV level. (**e**) Papillary muscle level. (**f**) Apex level. *Abbreviations*: *RVOT* right ventricular outflow tract, *Ao* aorta, *mPA* main pulmonary artery, *RPA* and *LPA* right and left pulmonary arteries, *RA* right atrium *LA* left atrium, *RCC, LCC* and *NCC* right, left and non-coronary cusps of aortic valve, *RV* right ventricle, *IVS* interventricular septum, *AMVL* and *PMVL* anterior and posterior mitral valve leaflets, *LV* left ventricle

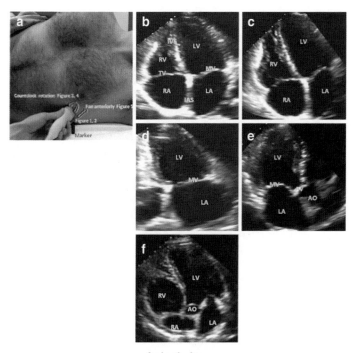

Apical view

FIGURE 2.5 Transducer position and echocardiographic images for apical views. (**a**) Probe position. (**b**) Apex 4-chamber view. (**c**) RV focused 4-chamber view. (**d**) Apex 2-chamber view. (**e**) Apex 3-chamber view. (**f**) Apex 5-chamber view. *Abbreviations. LA* and *RA* left and right atria, *LV* and *RV* left and right ventricles, *ias* and *ivs* interatrial and interventricular septi, *AMVL* and *PMVL* anterior and posterior mitral valve leaflets, *ATVL* and *PTVL* anteropr and posterior tricuspid valve leaflets, *MV* mitral valve, *AV* aortic valve, *AO* aorta

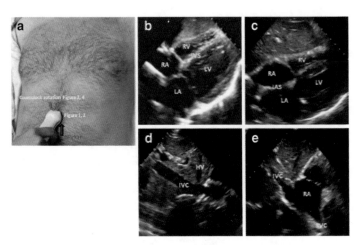

Subcostal view

FIGURE 2.6 Transducer position and echocardiographic images for subcostal views. (**a**) Probe position. (**b**) 1, 4-chamber view. (**c**) 2, 4-chamber view. (**d**) IVC view. (**e**) Bi-caval view. *Abbreviations*: LA and *RA* left and right ventricles, *LV* and *RV* left and right ventricles, *IVS* interventricular septum, *IAS* interatrial septum, *IVC* inferior vena cava, *HV* hepatic vein, *SVC* superior vena cava

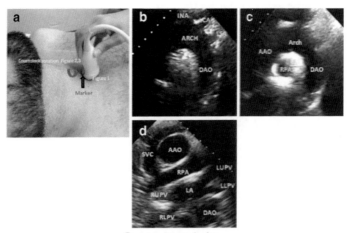

Suprasternal view

Figure 2.7 Transducer position and echocardiographic images for suprasternal views. (**a**) Probe position. (**b**) Suprasternal long-axis view. (**c**) Suprasternal long-axis view. (**d**) Suprasternal short-axis view. *Abbreviations*: *DAO* descending aorta, *IA* innominate artery, *LCA* left subclavian artery, *LCA* left carotid artery, *AAO* ascending aorta, *RPA* right pulmonary artery, *RUPV, RLPV, LUPV* and *RLPV* right upper, right lower, left upper and left lower pulmonary veins, *SVC* superio vena cava, *DAO* descending aorta, *LA* left atrium

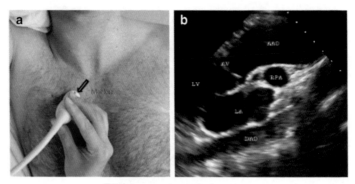

Right parasternal views

FIGURE 2.8 Transducer position and echocardiographic images for right suprasternal view. (**a**) Probe position. (**b**) Right parasternal view. *Abbreviation*: *LA* and *LV* left atria and ventricle, *AV* aortic valve, *AAO* and *DAO* ascending and descending aorta, *RPA* right pulmonary artery

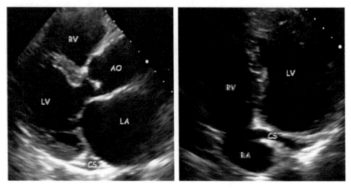

Coronary sinus

FIGURE 2.9 Parasternal long axis (*left*) and modified apical (*right*) views used to image coronary sinus. *Abbreviations*: *CS* coronary sinus, *LA* and *LV* left atrium and ventricle, *RA* and *RV* right atrium and ventricle, *Ao* aorta

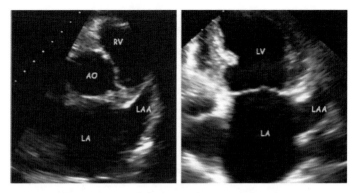

LA appendage

FIGURE 2.10 Parasternal short axis (*left*) and apical two chamber (*right*) views showing left atrial appendage (*LAA*). *Abbreviations: LA* left atrium, *LV* left ventricle, *RV* right ventricle, *AO* aorta

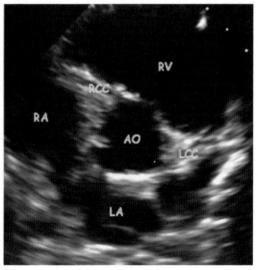

Coronary arteries

FIGURE 2.11 Parasternal short axis view showing coronary arteries. *Abbreviations: LCC* and *RCC* left and right coronary arteries, *LA* and *RA* left and right atrium, *RV* right ventricle, *AO* aorta

Interesting fact: The names behind the structures

Eustachian valve – was first described by sixteenth century Italian anatomist Bartolomeo Eustachi who is also famous for discovering adrenal gland, rediscovering Eustachean tube, describing the internal and anterior muscles of the malleus and stapedius along with figure of the cochlea, discovery of thorasic duct and many other structures [1].

Chiari network – first described by Austrian pathologist Hans Chiari in 1897. He is also famous for describing along with co-authors Arnold-Chiari malformation and Budd Chiari syndrome [2].

The Thebesian valve, a caudal remnant of the embryonic sinoatrial valves which is guarding coronary sinus, was originally described by Silesian physician Adam Christian Thebesius more than 300 years ago. He is also famous for describing venous tributaries which drain directly into cardiac chambers (in his graduate thesis, De circulo sangunis in corde (On the Circulation of the Blood in the Heart), 1708) [3].

References

1. Lariaux DL. Bartolomeo Eustachi (Eaustachius)(1520-1574). Endocrinologist. 2007;17(4):195.
2. Tubbs RS, Cohen-Gadol AA. Hans Chiari (1851-1916). J Neurol. 2010;257(7):1218–20.
3. Loukas M, Clarke P, Tubbs RS, Kolbinger W. Adam Christian Thebesius, a historical perspective. Int J Cardiol. 2008;129(1): 138–40.

Chapter 3
Chamber Dimensions

Dmitriy Kireyev and Judy Hung

Abbreviations

d	Diastole
LVIDd	Left Ventricular Internal Dimension end-diastole
LVIDs	Left Ventricular Internal Dimension end-systole
PWT	Posterior Wall Thickness
RVOT	Right Ventricular Outflow Tract
RWT	Relative wall thickness
s	Systole
SWT	Septal wall thickness

D. Kireyev, MD (✉) • J. Hung, MD
Echocardiography, Division of Cardiology,
Massachusetts General Hospital, Boston, MA, USA
e-mail: dimonk5@yahoo.com;
JHUNG@mgh.harvard.edu

D. Kireyev, J. Hung (eds.), *Cardiac Imaging in Clinical
Practice*, In Clinical Practice,
DOI 10.1007/978-3-319-21458-0_3,
© Springer International Publishing Switzerland 2016

Determination of End Systole/End Diastole

End Systole is determined by either:

- one frame before mitral valve opening
  or
- frame in which LV has a smallest dimension
  or
- end of T wave

End Diastole is determined by either:

- one frame after mitral valve closure
  or
- frame in which LV dimension is largest
  or
- onset of QRS complex

Left Ventricle

Obtain measurements:

- Posterior and Septal Wall Thickness measured at end diastole
- Parasternal long axis view: at mitral valve leaflet tips
- Parasternal short axis view: at mitral chordae level
- Measure tissue-blood interface for LVIDd and LVIDs

Linear dimensions [1–3]
Men

	Normal	Mildly enlarged	Moderately enlarged	Severely enlarged
LVEDD (cm)	4.2–5.8	5.9–6.3	6.4–6.8	>6.8
LVEDD/ BSA(cm/m^2)	2.2–3.0	3.1–3.3	3.4–3.6	>3.6
LVESD (cm)	2.5–4.0	4.1–4.3	4.4–4.5	>4.5

	Normal	Mildly enlarged	Moderately enlarged	Severely enlarged
LVESD/BSA (cm/m^2)	1.3–2.1	2.2–2.3	2.4–2.5	>2.6
Septal/ posterior wall thickness(cm)	0.6–1.0	1.1–1.3	1.4–1.6	≥1.6

Women

	Normal	Mildly enlarged	Moderately enlarged	Severely enlarged
LVEDD (cm)	3.8–5.2	5.3–5.6	5.7–6.1	>6.1
LVEDD/ BSA(cm/m^2)	2.3–3.1	3.2–3.4	3.5–3.7	>3.7
LVESD (cm)	2.2–3.5	3.6–3.8	3.9–4.1	>4.1
LVESD/BSA (cm/m^2)	1.3–2.1	2.2–2.3	2.4–2.6	>2.6
Septal/ posterior wall thickness(cm)	0.6–0.9	1.0–1.2	1.3–1.5	≥1.5

LV Function

– linear dimension method (Fig. 3.1)
– biplane method of disks (Fig. 3.2)

Left ventricular systolic function parameters [3]

	Normal	Mildly decreased	Moderately enlarged	Severely decreased
Ejection fraction (%)				
Men	52–74	41–51	30–40	<30
Women	54–74	41–53	30–40	<30

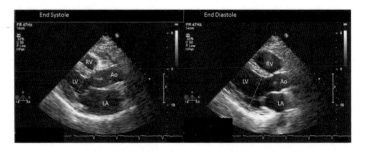

FIGURE 3.1 left panel: parasternal long axis view end-systole; right panel: parasternal long axis view end-diastole. LV internal dimensions (*green line*) are measured at mitral leaflet tips. The posterior wall (PW) and septal wall (SW) thickness are measured at end diastole. *LA* left atrium, *LV* left ventricle, *RV* right ventricle, *Ao* aorta

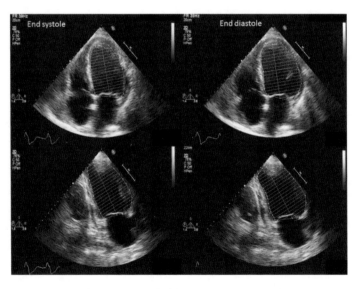

FIGURE 3.2 Biplane method of disks method of measuring LVEF. The *left column* shows end systolic apical four and two chamber views, respectively. The *right column* shows end diastolic apical and four chamber views

Left Atrium

- measure in end systole
- exclude pulmonary veins and atrial appendage
- measure anterior-posterior dimension from parasternal long axis view (Fig. 3.3)
- LA volume can be measured by area-length or biplane method of discs is recommended method

Area-Length Method (Fig. 3.4):

$$V_{LA} = 8/3\pi \cdot A_1 \cdot A_2 / L$$

where A1, A2 – areas of LA from 4 and 2 chamber views, L – length (choose a shorter vertical diameter (mid mitral annulus to superior axis of LA) between 4 and 2 chamber views).

Or

Biplane Method of Discs (Simpson's rule method) (preferred) in Apical 4 and Apical 2 chamber method

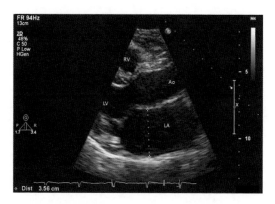

FIGURE 3.3 Parasternal long axis view – measurement of anterior-posterior dimension of left atrium performed at end-systole. *LA* left atrium, *LV* left ventricle, *RV* right ventricle, *Ao* aorta

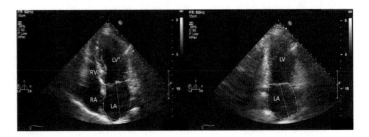

FIGURE 3.4 Apical four (*left*) and two chamber (*right*) views are used for left atrial volume calculation. *LA* left atrium, *LV* left ventricle, *RV* right ventricle, *RA* right atrium

Left atrial measurements [2, 4]
Men

	Normal	Mildly enlarged	Moderately enlarged	Severely enlarged
LA				
LA diameter (cm)	3.0–4.0	4.1–4.6	4.7–5.2	≥5.2
LA diameter/ BSA	1.5–2.3	2.4–2.6	2.7–2.9	≥3.0
LA area	≤20	20–30	30–40	≥40
LA volume (ml)	18–58	59–68	69–78	≥79
LA volume/ BSA (2015 guidelines)	16–34	35–41	42–48	>48

Women

	Normal	Mildly enlarged	Moderately enlarged	Severely enlarged
LA				
LA diameter (cm)	2.7–3.8	3.9–4.2	4.3–4.6	≥4.7
LA diameter/ BSA	1.5–2.3	2.4–2.6	2.7–2.9	≥3.0

	Normal	Mildly enlarged	Moderately enlarged	Severely enlarged
LA area	≤20	20–30	30–40	≥40
LA volume (ml)	22–52	53–62	63–72	≥73
LA volume/ BSA (2015 guidelines)	16–34	35–41	42–48	>48

Antero-posterior dimension (cm)[3]: men 3.0–4.0; women 2.7–3.8 cm

Right Ventricle

RV Size

- measure in end-diastole
- use 4 chamber view
- try to get RV-focused view
- RV should appear <2/3 of LV
- measure basal, mid-cavity and longitudinal dimensions (Fig. 3.5).

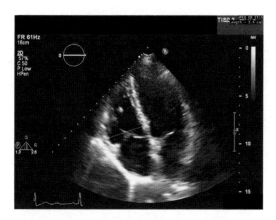

FIGURE 3.5 Right ventricular basal diameter measurement

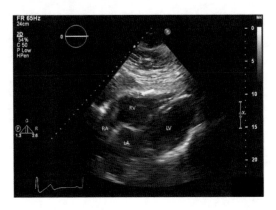

FIGURE 3.6 Measurement of RV wall thickness in subcostal view. *LA* left atrium, *LV* left ventricle, *RV* right ventricle, *RA* right atrium

Upper limits of normal [3, 5]
RV basal – 4.2 cm
RV mid-cavitary – 3.5 cm
Longitudinal dimension – 8.6 cm

RV Thickness [3, 5, 6]

– measure in end-diastole (Fig. 3.6)
– subcostal view
– exclude RV trabeculations, papillary muscles and epicardial fat

RV thickness upper limit of normal is 0.5 cm

RV Function

1. TAPSE (Fig. 3.7)

   – measures systolic movement of base of RV free wall
   – measures only one area of RV
   – TAPSE < 1.6 cm is abnormal [3]

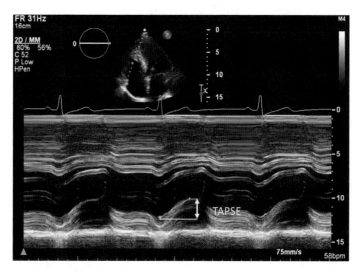

FIGURE 3.7 Tricuspid annular plane systolic excursion (*TAPSE*) measurement (*arrow*)

2. Tissue Doppler imaging

   – Tricuspid annulus and basal free wall can be assessed.
   – Limited data in elderly
   – S' < 10 cm/s is abnormal [3]
   – Color coded Doppler S' is lower (uses mean velocities)

3. 2D fractional area change: (end diastolic area-end systolic area)/end diastolic area 100 %

   – RV FAC < 35 % is abnormal [5]

4. RIMP – Myocardial performance index (or Tei index). MPI = isovolumic time/ejection time
   Pulsed Doppler vs. tissue Doppler methods

   – Doppler method: measure time (T1) from tricuspid valve opening to closing (either by tricuspid jet – onset to end or tricuspid inflow – end of A wave to beginning of E), ejection time (ET) – measure in RVOT (onset to cessation of flow). MPI = (T1-ET)/ET. Note: need

similar RR intervals since measurements are in different cycles – thus does not work well in irregular rhythms such as atrial fibrillation.
– Tissue Doppler method – all time intervals are obtained in single beat (please see picture below) [5]
– Normal values: MPI by Doppler method >0.43, MPI by pulsed tissue Doppler method >0.54 [3]

Right Atrium

RA Size

– Measure in end systole when atrium is largest (Fig. 3.8)
– Use 4 chamber view
– Long axis: mid tricuspid annulus to center of superior RA wall, short axis – mid portion of RA perpendicular to long axis
– Upper limits of normal [5]

Long axis 5.3 cm
Short axis 4.4 cm
Area 18 cm^2

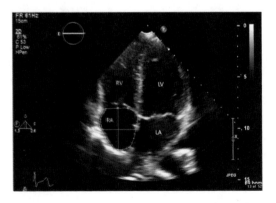

FIGURE 3.8 Apical four chamber view showing right atrial area and dimension measurements performed at end-systole. *LA* left atrium, *LV* left ventricle, *RV* right ventricle, *RA* right atrium

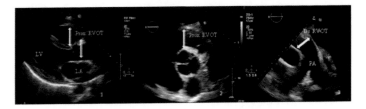

FIGURE 3.9 Parasternal long (*1*), and short (*2, 3*) axis views showing the measurement of Rights Ventricular Outflow Tract (*RVOT*) dimensions. *PA* pulmonary artery, *LA* left atrium, *LV* left ventricle

– RA volume indexes measured by single plane method of disks are mentioned in 2015 guidelines, but strict cutoffs still need to be defined.

Right Ventricular Outflow Tract (Fig. 3.9)

– Measure in end diastole on QRS deflection
– Parasternal short axis view proximal to pulmonary annulus is most reproducible
– Upper limits of normal:

Parasternal long axis view – 3.3 cm
Parasternal short axis view (distal) – 2.7 cm
Parasternal short axis view (proximal) – 3.5 cm

References

1. Ilercil A, O'Grady MJ, Roman MJ, Paranicas M, Lee ET, Welty TK, Fabsitz RR, Howard BV, Devereux RB. Reference values for echocardiographic measurements in urban and rural populations of differing ethnicity: the Strong Heart Study. J Am Soc Echocardiogr. 2001;14(6):601–11.
2. Lang RM, Bierig M, Devereux RB, Flachskampf FA, Foster E, Pellikka PA, Picard MH, Roman MJ, Seward J, Shanewise JS, Solomon SD, Spencer KT, Sutton MS, Stewart WJ, Chamber Quantification Writing Group; American Society of

Echocardiography's Guidelines and Standards Committee; European Association of Echocardiography. Recommendations for chamber quantification: a report from the American Society of Echocardiography's Guidelines and Standards Committee and the Chamber Quantification Writing Group, developed in conjunction with the European Association of Echocardiography, a branch of the European Society of Cardiology. J Am Soc Echocardiogr. 2005;18(12):1440–63.

3. Lang RM, Bierig M, Devereux RB, Flachskampf FA, Foster E, Pellikka PA, Picard MH, Roman MJ, Seward J, Shanewise J, Solomon S, Spencer KT, St John Sutton M, Stewart W, American Society of Echocardiography's Nomenclature and Standards Committee; Task Force on Chamber Quantification; American College of Cardiology Echocardiography Committee; American Heart Association; European Association of Echocardiography, European Society of Cardiology. Recommendations for chamber quantification. Eur J Echocardiogr. 2006;7(2):79–108.

4. Lang RM, Badano LP, Mor-Avi V, Afilalo J, Amrstrong A, et al. Recommendations for cardiac chamber quantification by echocardiography in adults. An update from the American Society of Echocardiography and the European Association of Cardiovascular imaging. J Am Soc Echocardiogr. 2015;28:1–39.

5. Rudski LG, Lai WW, Afilalo J, Hua L, Handschumacher MD, Chandrasekaran K, Solomon SD, Louie EK, Schiller NB. Guidelines for the echocardiographic assessment of the right heart in adults: a report from the American Society of Echocardiography endorsed by the European Association of Echocardiography, a registered branch of the European Society of Cardiology, and the Canadian Society of Echocardiography. J Am Soc Echocardiogr. 2010;23(7):685–713.

6. Matsukubo H, Matsuura T, Endo N, Asayama J, Watanabe T. Echocardiographic measurement of right ventricular wall thickness. A new application of subxiphoid echocardiography. Circulation. 1977;56(2):278–84.

Chapter 4
Valvular Quantification

Dmitriy Kireyev and Judy Hung

Echocardiography is the primary imaging modality to assess valvular quantification such as degree of valve stenosis and regurgitation as well as pressures in cardiac chambers. Flow velocities across valves and cardiac chambers can be measured using Doppler echocardiography.

Flow velocities can then be converted to pressure using the modified Bernoulli equation (Fig. 4.1). This is the basis for much of valvular quantification and cardiac chamber pressures.

The modified Bernoulli equation is derived from the Bernoulli equation which relates pressure drop as fluid speed changes across a tube due to change in diameter of the tube. This pressure drop has been applied to stenotic and regurgitant valve orifices to measure pressures across the valves.

$$\Delta P = \frac{1}{2}\rho\left(V_2^2 - V_1^2\right) + \rho\int\frac{dv}{dt}ds + R\left(\mu, V\right)$$

Electronic supplementary material The online version of this chapter (doi:10.1007/978-3-319-21458-0_4) contains supplementary material, which is available to authorized users.

D. Kireyev, MD (✉) • J. Hung, MD
Echocardiography, Division of Cardiology, Massachusetts General Hospital, Boston, MA, USA
e-mail: dimonk5@yahoo.com; JHUNG@mgh.harvard.edu

D. Kireyev, J. Hung (eds.), *Cardiac Imaging in Clinical Practice*, In Clinical Practice,
DOI 10.1007/978-3-319-21458-0_4,
© Springer International Publishing Switzerland 2016

Bernoulli Equation

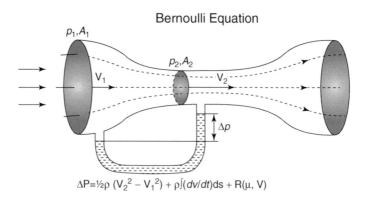

$$\Delta P = \tfrac{1}{2}\rho\,(V_2{}^2 - V_1{}^2) + \rho\!\int(dv/dt)ds + R(\mu, V)$$

Figure 4.1 illustrates the principle of Bernoulli Equation which relates pressure drop that occurs with changing fluid speeds across a narrowing in tube

where ρ is density of blood, V_1 and V_2 represents velocity proximal and distal to stenosis respectively. The second and third parts of the equation representing flow acceleration and viscous resistance components are usually relatively small and ignored in clinical practice [1].

The origin of 4 in modified Bernoulli equation:

Since we measure pressure in mmHg instead of Pascals, and the density of blood is approximately 1060 kg/m3, we get P (in Pa) = ½ · 0.0075 mmHg/Pa (conversion factor) · 1060 kg/m3 · (V22 – V12 (in m/s)) = 3.975 · (V22 – V12). (note: density of blood and conversion factors are approximated). Since 3.975 is close to 4, the equation is further modified to:

$$\Delta P = 4\left(V_2{}^2 - V_1{}^2\right) = \text{Modified Bernoulli Equation.}$$

For clinically important transvalvular gradients where V_2 is generally much greater than V_1, the $4\,V_1{}^2$ term is negligible compared to the $4\,V_2{}^2$ term and the $4\,V_1{}^2$ term is dropped further simplifying the equation to:

$$\Delta P = 4V_2{}^2 \text{ which is known as the simplified Bernoulli Equation.}$$

Things to remember:

- If $V_1 > 1.5$ m/s or $V_2 < 3$ m/s, then need to include the $4\,V_1^2$ term in the Bernoulli equation.
- Pressure recovery: determination of pressure gradient by CV Doppler assumes that all the energy which is transferred to kinetic energy of accelerated flow is dissipated completely and not recovered. The pressure recovery depends on both the effective orifice size of AS jet and aortic size.

More than you wanted to know :
Correction factor for pressure recovery :

$$P \approx 4(\upsilon_1^2 - \upsilon_0^2)(1-C)\; Where\; C$$

$$= 2\left(\frac{Effective\; orifice\; area}{Aortic\; Area} - \left(\frac{Effective\; orifice\; area}{Aortic\; Area} \right)^2 \right).$$

Aortic Stenosis

Transvalvular Pressures

Transvalvular pressures are estimated from velocities obtained by Doppler using the Simplified Bernoulli equation: $4\,V^2$ where V is the peak velocity (Fig. 4.2)

- Mean trans AV gradients are based on averaging of instantaneous gradients. In cases where $V_{prox} > 1.5$ m/s or $V_{distal} < 3$ m/s, it is recommended to use maximal gradients and velocities for stenosis severity estimation as mean gradients are often not accurately assessed [2].
- Maximal pressure gradient calculated is representing maximal transvalvular gradient, not peak LV to peak aortic difference which is obtained from cardiac catheterization (note the peak pressures are not simultaneous). Mean gradients should be used to compare gradients obtained by Doppler echocardiography to cardiac catheterization gradients [3].

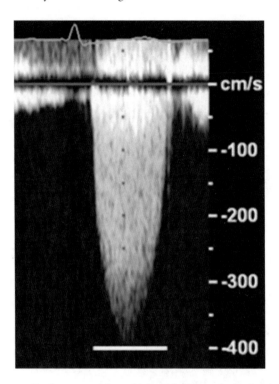

FIGURE 4.2 Peak transaortic velocity of 400 cm/s or 4 m/s (*solid white line*) as obtained by Doppler echocardiography in a patient with aortic stenosis; Peak pressure across the stenotic aortic valve can then be calculated as 4 (4 m/s)^2 = 64 mmHg

Aortic Valve Area Calculations

Aortic valve area in aortic stenosis is calculated using the continuity equation (Fig. 4.3). By the law of conservation of mass the volume flow is constant. Flow proximal to stenosis must equal flow distal to stenosis. Flow is calculated as cross sectional area times velocity and aortic valve area can be calculated as:

Aortic Valve Area Calculation by continuity equation

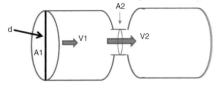

$$Flow = A1*V1 = A2*V2$$

$$A2 = (A1*V1) \div V2$$

A1 = (πr^2); r = d/2   V1   V2

FIGURE 4.3 illustrates continuity equation which is used to calculate aortic valve area in aortic stenosis. Flow proximal (Q1) to stenosis must equal flow distal (Q2) to stenosis by principle of conservation of mass. Flow is calculated as cross sectional area times velocity. A1 is the cross sectional area of the LVOT velocity and is calculated as πr^2 where r = d/2 and d is the diameter of the LVOT; V1 = proximal time velocity integral by pulse wave Doppler; V2 = maximum instantaneous time velocity integral across aortic valve by continuous wave Doppler

$$AVA \cdot VTI_{(AV)} = LVOT\,Area \cdot VTI_{(LVOT)}$$

$$Thus\,AVA = \frac{LVOT\,Area \cdot VTI(LVOT)}{VTI(AV)}$$

$$= \frac{\pi D(LVOT)^2/4 \cdot VTI(LVOT)}{VTI(AV)}$$

$$\approx \frac{0.785\,D(LVOT)^2 \cdot VTI(LVOT)}{VTI(AV)}$$

$$\text{Or similarly } AVA = \frac{0.785\,D(LVOT)^2 \cdot (LVOT)}{(AV)}$$

Points to remember:

- The shape of LVOT is not circular but elliptical in many patients and thus the AVA calculation is often underestimated
- The actual calculated area is effective orifice area, not the anatomical valve area (and thus is smaller).
- Pliability and shape inlet to the valve orifice will affect location and size of vena contracta
- Peak velocities of LVOT and aortic valve can be substituted for time velocity integral

Dimensionless Index

- $v_{LVOT}/v_{AorticValve} \leq 0.25$ is sensitive determination of severity of aortic stenosis in both normal and low cardiac output conditions [4].
- Ratio needs to be interpreted with caution in patients with coexistent Aortic Regurgitation which is moderate or severe [5].

Mitral Valve Stenosis

Rheumatic Mitral Stenosis

Rheumatic mitral stenosis severity is assessed by valve area using direct planimetry of the mitral valve orifice or by pressure half time (PHT) or deceleration time (DT).

Direct Planimetry is preferred method if images are of good quality (Fig. 4.4). Planimetry is performed in the short axis view at the level of the smallest mitral valve orifice. This is generally determined by scanning back and forth to

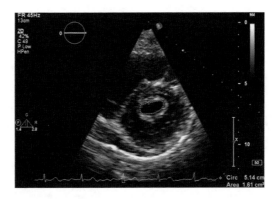

FIGURE 4.4 Direct planimetry of mitral valve area in patient with rheumatic mitral stenosis

determine the smallest orifice. 3D guided measurement of mitral valve area planimetry has been shown to improve reproducibility of MVA area measurements.

Pressure Half Time (PHT) or Deceleration Time (DT):

MVA can be calculated by using the following empirically derived formulas:

$MVA = 220 / PHT$ (Fig. 4.5) or $MVA = 750 / DT$. These are simple relatively reproducible measurements to MVA. However, one should use both formulas with caution since they do not take into consideration other variables such as initial pressure gradient, atrial and ventricular compliance, aortic regurgitation, etc [6]. With significant aortic regurgitation (moderate or greater) the MVA can be overestimated.

Mean transmitral gradients (Fig. 4.6) are important as confirmatory data to determine the severity of mitral stenosis. However it is important to consider that gradients are flow related and heart rate or cardiac output can impact the gradients. We recommend documenting heart rate when reporting the gradient.

Alternate methods for calculating mitral valve area are the Continuity equation and PISA (Proximal Isovelocity Surface Area) method. These latter two methods are time consuming and require significant operator experience. These methods are not applied widely in clinical laboratories.

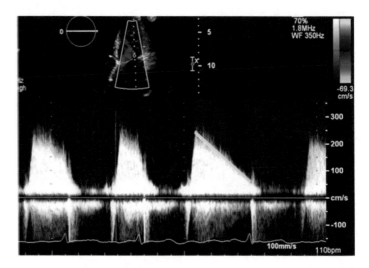

FIGURE 4.5 Measurement of pressure half time in patient with rheumatic mitral stenosis. PHT is measured by measuring deceleration slope of mitral gradient (*yellow line*)

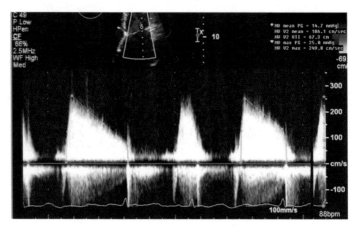

FIGURE 4.6 Measurement of peak and mean transmitral gradient

Continuity equation :

$$MVA = \pi \frac{D^2}{4} \times \frac{VTI\,(aortic)}{VTI\,(mitral)} \text{ where D is LVOT diameter}$$

It is important to remember that care needs to be taken in measuring LVOT diameter as both the echocardiographic cut angle and shape of LVOT (which becomes more elliptical further away from AV) are important sources of error.

PISA (Proximal Isovelocity Surface Area):

$$MVA = 2\pi R^2 \upsilon_{aliasing} / \upsilon_{max(mitral)} \cdot \alpha / 180$$

Not used frequently as this method is technically difficult, time consuming and assumes that isovelocity progression shapes are actually hemispherical in shape.

Calcific Mitral Stenosis

Calcific mitral stenosis results from degenerative valvular changes from annular calcification. Measurement of mitral area by direct planimetry is difficult in calcific MS due to the acoustic shadowing from the calcified mitral orifice. In addition, PHT is not validated for calcific mitral stenosis. Typically, transmitral gradients are used to assess severity of stenosis for calcific MS.

Tricuspid Valve Stenosis (Fig. 4.7; Video 4.1)

- Data is less robust than for aortic and mitral stenosis.
- Mean pressure gradient (≥5 mmHg) and time velocity integral (>60 cm) are more frequently used as an indicator of tricuspid stenosis.
- Tricuspid valve area approximated by 190/(pressure half time) is not as precise and suffers from limitations similar to evaluation of mitral valve area by pressure half time.

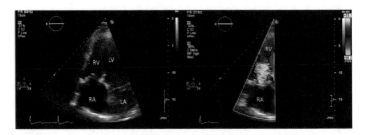

FIGURE 4.7 Apical four chamber view of patient with tricuspid stenosis. Notice the thickened valves on the left part of the image and color Doppler image showing turbulent flow through the valve in end diastole. *LA* left atrium, *LV* left ventricle, *RV* right ventricle, *RA* right atrium

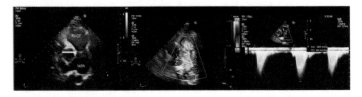

FIGURE 4.8 Patient with pulmonic stenosis. Notice the thickened pulmonic valve (*arrow*) on the *left panel*. The *middle panel* of the figure shows significant turbulence after consistent with stenotic flow. *Right panel* shows corresponding elevated gradients across the stenotic pulmonic valve. *MPA* main pulmonary artery

Pulmonic Valve Stenosis (Fig. 4.8)

Pulmonary stenosis is generally assessed by peak velocity and peak and mean transpulmonary gradients. Peak gradients >64 mmHg indicate severe pulmonary stenosis.

Aortic Valve Regurgitation
(Figs. 4.9, 4.10, and 4.11)

Grading of aortic regurgitation is primarily based on color Doppler techniques as described below.

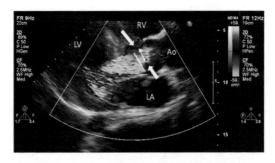

FIGURE 4.9 Left panel shows color Doppler image of aortic regurgitant jet in parasternal long axis view. Vena contracta is narrowest portion of jet as the level of the aortic leaflets (*arrows*); Proximal jet width is width of jet just as it exits the leaflets and enters the LVOT (*solid line*). *LA* left atrium, *LV* left ventricle, *RV* right ventricle, *Ao* aorta

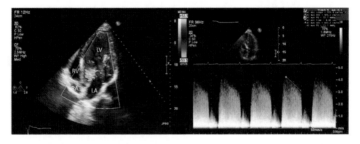

FIGURE 4.10 Pressure half time of aortic regurgitant flow. *LA* left atrium, *LV* left ventricle, *RV* right ventricle, *RA* right atrium

(a) Width of regurgitant jet relative to LVOT width (Fig. 4.9; Video 4.2)

Maximal proximal jet width/LVOT diameter from parasternal long axis view and cross sectional area of the jet/cross sectional area of LVOT

Multiple points need to be taken into consideration; jet direction, eccentricity, color gain, pulse repetition frequency, blood pressure at the time of measurement

(b) Vena contracta (Fig. 4.9)

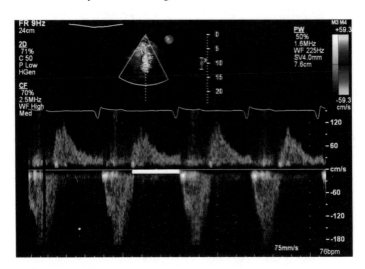

FIGURE 4.11 Diastolic flow reversal in the descending thoracic aorta (*white line*)

Smallest area of the flow, effective regurgitant orifice area (EROA) approximation. Remember: it is SMALLER than actual anatomic regurgitant area. If the orifice size is rigid, vena contracta is independent of flow rate and pressure difference between LA and LV.

Limitations: multiple jets, irregular jet shape, pliable valve (which changes area based on pressure difference or cardiac output)

(c) Proximal Isovelocity Surface Area [7]

$$EROA = 2\pi R^2 \frac{\upsilon_{aliasing}}{\upsilon_{max(ar)}}$$

Technically demanding method; requires operator experience. Flow convergence radius should be measured in early diastole.

(d) Regurgitant volume and fraction: both are technically demanding with potential sourced of error in measurements of LVOT and MV diameters as well as VTIs [7]

Regurgitant Volume:

$$RV = EROA \cdot VTI_{AR}$$

$$RV = \frac{\pi}{4}\left(LVOT\,D\right)^2 \cdot VTI_{Ao} - \frac{\pi}{4}\left(MV\,D\right)^2 \cdot VTI_{MV}$$

$$RV = Stroke\,V - \frac{\pi}{4}\left(MV\,D\right)^2 \cdot VTI_{MV}$$

Regurgitant Fraction:

$$RF = RV\,/\,SV = RV\,/\left(\frac{\pi}{4}\left(LVOT\,D\right)^2 \cdot VTI_{Ao}\right)$$

(e) Diastolic pressure half time (Fig. 4.10)

PHT is relatively easy to measure. However, LV diastolic pressure and compliance can significantly alter this parameter.

(f) Diastolic flow reversal in the descending thoracic or abdominal aorta (Fig. 4.11)

Usually associated with severe AR

Mitral Regurgitation

(a) Distal regurgitant jet area (Fig. 4.12; Video 4.3)
   - presented as ratio distal jet area divided by left atrial area
   - measured in apical views
   - eccentric jets are underestimated by jet area method
   - loading (blood pressure, volume status) and machine settings (color gain) affect size of MR jet

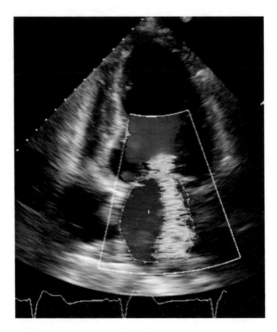

FIGURE 4.12 Distal jet area is traced at its maximal point in systole and divided by left atrial area in same frame

(b) Vena contracta (Fig. 4.13)
 – Parasternal long axis view is preferred view to measure
 – Two chamber view should not be used as it overestimates vena contracta size.
 – narrow range for MR grading, thus small measurement differences can change grade of MR category; important to maximize resolution (ZOOM)

(c) Proximal Isovelocity Surface Area Method: Quantitates mitral regurgitation by calculating an effective regurgitant orifice area, mitral regurgitant volume and regurgitant fraction (Fig. 4.14)

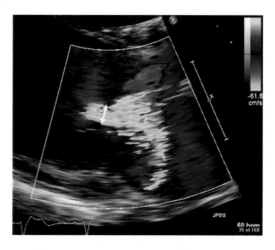

FIGURE 4.13 Color Doppler image of vena contracta region in parasternal long axis view. Vena contracta is narrowest width of color jet at the level of the leaflets (*white arrow*)

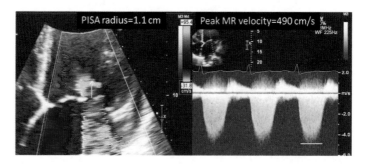

FIGURE 4.14 *Left panel* shows magnified image of PISA zone which has been baseline shifted toward direction of jet to an aliasing velocity of 31.8 cm/s (*square box*). The PISA radius is measured from top of hemispherical shell to end of shell and measures 1.1 cm (*white line*). *Right panel* shows peak veocity of MR jet is 490 cm/s. Calculating EROA formula yields:

$$EROA = 3.14(1.1 cm)^2 (31.8 cm/s) \div 490 cm/s = 0.49 cm^2$$

$$EROA = 2\pi R^2 \frac{\upsilon aliasing}{\upsilon max(MR)} \text{ where R is the radius of the PISA zone}$$

Regurgitant Volume:

$$RV = EROA \cdot VTI_{MR}$$

$$RV = \frac{\pi}{4}(MV\,D)^2 \cdot VTI_{MV} - \frac{\pi}{4}(LVOT\,D)^2 \cdot VTI_{MV}$$

$$RV = Stroke\,V - \frac{\pi}{4}(MV\,D)^2 \cdot VTI_{MV}$$

Regurgitant Fraction

$$RF = RV/SV = RV/\left(\frac{\pi}{4}(MV\,D)^2 \cdot VTI_{MV}\right)$$

- technically demanding
- magnify PISA region (ZOOM)
- baseline shift toward direction of flow
- PISA radius measured in mid-late systole

Tricuspid Regurgitation

(a) Size of regurgitant jet (Fig. 4.15; Video 4.4)

- Most common method to measure TR
- Can be expressed as absolute jet area or as ratio of jet area/right atrial area
- Measured in apical views

(b) Vena contracta (Fig. 4.16)

- Measured in apical four chamber view or parasternal short axis view
- Is more reliable than regurgitant jet area and correlates well with EROA
- Values of 0.7 cm is associated with severe TR

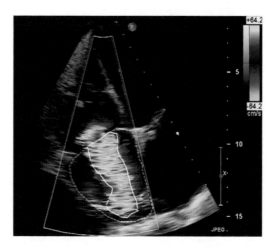

FIGURE 4.15 Apical four chamber view showing severe TR. Distal jet area (*solid line*) is traced at its maximal point in systole and divided by right atrial area in same frame (*Dashed lines*)

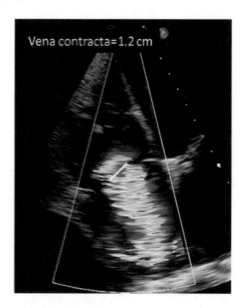

FIGURE 4.16 Vena contracta measurement of 1.2 cm (*solid line*) is consistent with severe TR

(c) Proximal Isovelocity Surface Area

Calculates an effective regurgitant orifice area :

$$EROA = 2\pi R^2 \frac{\upsilon \text{aliasing}}{\upsilon \text{max}(TR)}$$

- Technically demanding method and not well validated for TR

(d) Systolic flow reversal in hepatic vein (Fig. 4.17). Usually associated with severe TR.

Pulmonic Regurgitation

- Quantitative variables to measure PR are less validated than for other regurgitant valve lesions
- Semi quantitative measure is ratio of jet width or area to RVOT width or area (Fig. 4.18)
- Pressure half time is measured from the initial peak of the continuous wave tracing of the PR jet (Fig. 4.19) and values of <100 ms are consistent with severe PR

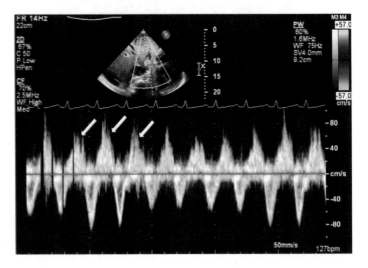

FIGURE 4.17 Holosystolic flow reversal (*arrows*) in hepatic vein in a patient with severe TR

- Fast deceleration time or laminar Doppler flow profile is c/w severe PR. A deceleration time of less 260 ms is c/w severe PR.

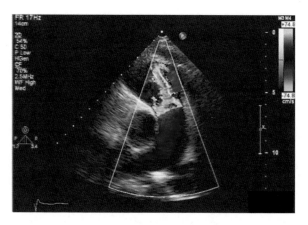

FIGURE 4.18 Color Doppler images in parasternal short axis view showing a wide jet of severe pulmonic regurgitation occupying almost the whole width of RVOT

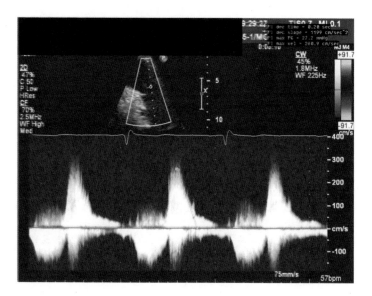

FIGURE 4.19 Pressure half time is measured from the initial peak of the continuous wave tracing of the PR jet

References

1. Baumgartner H, Hung J, Bermejo J, Chambers JB, Evangelista A, Griffin BP, Iung B, Otto CM, Pellikka PA, Quiñones M, American Society of Echocardiography; European Association of Echocardiography. Echocardiographic assessment of valve stenosis: EAE/ASE recommendations for clinical practice. J Am Soc Echocardiogr. 2009;22(1):1–23.
2. Baumgartner H, Kratzer H, Helmreich G, Kuehn P. Determination of aortic valve area by Doppler echocardiography using the continuity equation: a critical evaluation. Cardiology. 1990;77(2): 101–11.
3. Oh JK, Taliercio CP, Holmes Jr DR, Reeder GS, Bailey KR, Seward JB, Tajik AJ. Prediction of the severity of aortic stenosis by Doppler aortic valve area determination: prospective Doppler-catheterization correlation in 100 patients. J Am Coll Cardiol. 1988;11(6):1227–34.
4. Otto CM, Pearlman AS, Comess KA, Reamer RP, Janko CL, Huntsman LL. Determination of the stenotic aortic valve area in adults using Doppler echocardiography. J Am Coll Cardiol. 1986;7(3):509–17.
5. Thomas JD, Weyman AE. Doppler mitral pressure half-time: a clinical tool in search of theoretical justification. J Am Coll Cardiol. 1987;10(4):923–9.
6. Zoghbi WA, Enriquez-Sarano M, Foster E, Grayburn PA, Kraft CD, Levine RA, Nihoyannopoulos P, Otto CM, Quinones MA, Rakowski H, Stewart WJ, Waggoner A, Weissman NJ, American Society of Echocardiography. Recommendations for evaluation of the severity of native valvular regurgitation with two-dimensional and Doppler echocardiography. J Am Soc Echocardiogr. 2003;16(7):777–802.
7. Grossmann G, Stein M, Kochs M, Höher M, Koenig W, Hombach V, Giesler M. Comparison of the proximal flow convergence method and the jet area method for the assessment of the severity of tricuspid regurgitation. Eur Heart J. 1998;19(4):652–9.

Chapter 5
Valvular Pathology

Dmitriy Kireyev and Judy Hung

Aortic Valve Lesions

Aortic Stenosis (Videos 5.1, 5.2, 5.3, and 5.4)

Etiology

1. Calcific stenosis of tricuspid valve (Fig. 5.1)
2. Calcific stenosis of congenitally abnormal valve – review of 932 excised aortic valves (in patients without concomitant mitral valve replacement or mitral stenosis) showed that 59 % of men and 46 % of women had bicuspid or unicuspid aortic valve [1]

Electronic supplementary material The online version of this chapter (doi:10.1007/978-3-319-21458-0_5) contains supplementary material, which is available to authorized users.

D. Kireyev, MD (✉) • J. Hung, MD
Echocardiography, Division of Cardiology,
Massachusetts General Hospital, Boston, MA, USA
e-mail: dimonk5@yahoo.com; JHUNG@mgh.harvard.edu

D. Kireyev, J. Hung (eds.), *Cardiac Imaging in Clinical Practice*, In Clinical Practice,
DOI 10.1007/978-3-319-21458-0_5,
© Springer International Publishing Switzerland 2016

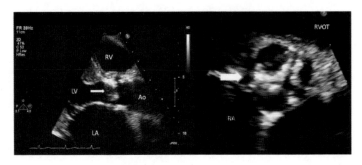

FIGURE 5.1 Calcified tricuspid aortic valve stenosis seen in long axis (*left*) and short axis (*right*); note significant leaflet calcification restriction of motion (*arrows*). *LA* left atrium, *LV* left ventricle, *RV* right ventricle, *Ao* aorta, *RA* right atrium

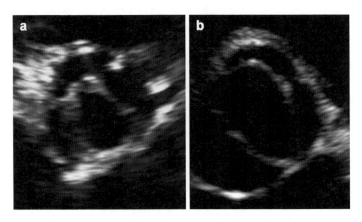

FIGURE 5.2 (**a**) Shows unicupsid aortic valve. (**b**) Shows bicuspid aortic valve with fusion of the right and left leaflets

Unicuspid aortic valve

- Anatomy: One leaflet; acommissural (no commissure) or unicommissural-one commissure (Fig. 5.2a)
- Rare form of congenital aortic stenosis (0.02 % incidence)

Bicuspid aortic valve (Fig. 5.2b)

- Anatomy: two leaflets and two commissures from cusp fusion of right and left – 86 %, cusp fusion of right and non-coronary – 12 %, left and non-coronary – 3 % [2]
- Associated lesions: coarctation of aorta, dilatation of aortic root, ascending aorta, sinus of Valsalva aneurysm, sub and supra valvular aortic stenosis, Shone's complex, Turners Syndrome, ventricular septal defect [3, 4].

3. Rheumatic heart disease
   Important etiology of aortic stenosis in developing countries

N.B. up to 80 % of patients with AS will also have AR

Interesting fact: First description and sketches of bicuspid aortic valve are attributed to Leonardo da Vinci [5]

Evaluation of Aortic Valve

- Morphology of the valve
- Aortic Stenosis velocity by continuous wave Doppler (note, the recorded velocity is at effective orifice area, not anatomic area) [6]. N.B. Measure maximal velocity at outer edge of dark signal
- Mean and maximal transaortic gradient (do not forget that $\Delta P = 4$ (V^2max–V^2proximal) for cases when proximal velocity is >1.5 m/s or aortic velocity is <1.5 m/s)
- LVOT diameter – measure in mid systole (N.B. in many patients LVOT is elliptical and not circular leading to underestimation of AVA)
- LVOT velocity by pulsed Doppler
- N.B. pressure recovery has to be taken into account for aortic size <30 mm (pressure drop across the stenosis will be overestimated)

$$AVA = AREA_{LVOT} \cdot VTI_{LVOT} / VTI_{AV} = p / 4 D^2_{LVOT} \cdot VTI_{LVOT} / VTI_{AV}$$

Aortic stenosis severity [7, 8]

	Mild	**Moderate**	**Severe**
AVA (cm^2)	>1.5	1.0–1.5	$\leq$1
AVA index (cm^2 /m^2)			$\leq$0.6
Mean Gradient (mm Hg)	<20	20–39	$\geq$40
Aortic Jet Velocity (m/s)	2.0–2.9	3.0–3.9	$\geq$4
Velocity Ratio (LVOT/AV)	>0.5	0.25–0.5	<0.25

Note: V < 2.5 m/s with normal cardiac output – aortic sclerosis

Low Flow Low Gradient Aortic Stenosis with decreased Ejection Fraction (present in 5–10 % of Severe AS patients) [9, 10]

– LVEF < 40 %
– Mean pressure gradient <30–40 mmHg
– Effective orifice area <1.0 cm^2

Possible situations: severe AS causing LV dysfunction limiting the ability to generate high transaortic valve gradients or patient with moderate AS and LV dysfunction from other etiology.

Dobutamine stress test:

– Get images at rest, 2.5–5 µg/kg/min, 10 µg/kg/min, 20 µg/kg/min (increase dose every 3–5 min)
– Record: LVOT diameter (at rest), AV VTI, LVOT VTI, AV mean pressure gradient, Aortic valve V$_{max}$, Heart Rate
– Stop when positive result is obtained or heart rate goes over 20 bpm over the baseline or exceeds 100 bpm, blood

pressure drops, or when there are appearances of arrhythmias or symptoms.

– Useful formulas:

$$AVA = \pi / 4 D^2_{LVOT} \cdot VTI_{LVOT} / VTI_{AV}$$
$$SV = \pi / 4 D^2_{LVOT} \cdot VTI_{LVOT}$$
$$CO = \pi / 4 D^2_{LVOT} \cdot VTI_{LVOT} \, HR$$

– Result interpretation [7]

(a) Vmax >4 m/s or mean pressure gradient >40 mmHg (assuming AVA <1 cm^2) – severe stenosis

(b) AVA >1 cm^2 – stenosis is not severe

(c) Evaluate contractile reserve (increase of stroke volume or cardiac output by >20 %). Note – does not predict improvement of EF, but predicts mortality [11, 12].

Aortic Regurgitation

Etiology

Aortic Root Dilatation (Secondary)

Marfan's syndrome
Idiopathic aortic dilation
Cystic medial necrosis
Senile aortic ectasia and dilation
Syphilitic aortitis
Giant cell arteritis
Takayasu's arteritis
Ankylosing spondylitis

Valvular Abnormalities (Primary)

Rheumatic fever
Infective endocarditis
Collagen vascular diseases
Degenerative aortic valve disease
Bicuspid Aortic Valve
Unicuspid Aortic Valve
Quadricuspid Aortic Valve (Fig. 5.3)

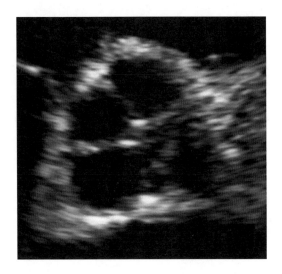

FIGURE 5.3 Quadricuspid aortic valve; all four leaflets best seen when valve is closed forming a characteristic cross sign

Evaluation

- Aortic valve morphology
- Aortic Root Morphology
- Left Ventricle (dimensions and performance)
- Aortic Flow
- Left ventricular size and function
- Flow in the aorta

Useful Formulas
- Deceleration time:

$$DT = 0.29\,PHT$$

- <u>Regurgitant Volume</u>

$$RV = EROA \cdot VTI_{AR}$$
$$RV = \pi/4\left(LVOT\,D\right)^2 \cdot VTI_{Ao} - \pi/4\left(MV\,D\right)^2 \cdot VTI_{MV}$$

$$RV = Stroke\,V - \pi/4\left(MV\,D\right)^2 \cdot VTI_{MV}$$

- Regurgitant Fraction

$$\mathbf{RF} = \mathbf{RV} / \mathbf{SV} = \mathbf{RV} / \left(\pi / 4 (\mathbf{LVOT\,D})^2 \cdot \mathbf{VTI}_{Ao} \right)$$

- EROA

$$\mathbf{EROA} = \mathbf{RV} / \mathbf{VTI}_{AR} \,; \mathbf{EROA} = 2\pi r^2 \upsilon_{aliasing} / \upsilon_{AR}$$

Chronic aortic regurgitation evaluation [8, 13]

	Mild	Moderate	Severe
Regurgitant Jet/ LVOT Diameter	<0.25	0.25–0.45 mild-moderate 0.46–0.64 mod-severe	>0.65
Regurgitant Jet Area/LVOT Area (cross sectional area)	<0.05	0.05–0.2 mild-moderate 0.21–0.59 moderate to severe	≥0.6
Regurgitant Volume (ml)	<30	30–44 mild-moderate 45–59 moderate to severe	≥60
Regurgitant fraction	<30 %	30–39 mild-moderate 40–49 moderate to severe	≥50 %
EROA (cm²)	<0.1	0.1–0.19 mild-moderate 0.2–0.29 mod-severe	≥0.3

(continued)

	Mild	Moderate	Severe
Vena Contracta (cm)	<0.3	0.3–0.6	>0.6
Pressure Half-time (ms) (=0.29DT)	>500		<200
Decceleration rate (m/s^2)	<2		>3.5
MV flow pattern			restrictive
Aortic Doppler	Mild early diastolic reversal in descending aorta		Holodiastolic flow reversal in descending aorta
Doppler	Faint continuous Doppler sign		Dense continuous Doppler sign
LVEDD (mm)	<55		>75

Mitral Valve Lesions

Mitral valve has such a name due to its resemblance to a mitre, a bishop's headgear [14].

Mitral Stenosis

Etiology

Rheumatic Heart Disease (vast majority of cases)
Congenital mitral stenosis
Severe calcification of mitral annulus
Systemic lupus erythematosus (rare)
Fabry's disease (rare)

Evaluation

– Mitral valve morphology
– Left Atrial size
– Pulmonary Pressures

Rheumatic Mitral Stenosis (Fig. 5.4, Videos 5.5 and 5.6)

- Doming of the tip "Hockey stick appearance" of anterior mitral leaflet (long axis view)
- Immobility of posterior leaflet
- "Fish mouth" appearance – short axis
- Diastolic mitral leaflet doming towards LA – only in rheumatic and congenital mitral stenosis

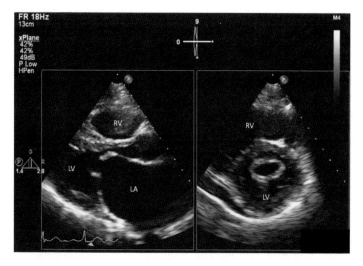

FIGURE 5.4 Parasternal long (*left*) and short axis (*right*) views showing rheumatic mitral stenosis. Note the hockey-stick appearance of the anterior leaflet (left image) consistent with rheumatic etiology of stenosis. Parasternal short axis view shows commissural fusion and "fish mouth" opening in rheumatic mitral stenosis. *LA* left atrium, *LV* left ventricle, *RV* right ventricle

Measurements

1. Planimetry – most precise if have good views
2. MVA = 220/PHT Note: $\upsilon = 0.7\ \upsilon_{max}$ at PHT
3. MVA = 750/DT
4. PISA: EROA = $2\pi r^2\ \upsilon_{aliasing}\ /\ \upsilon_{MR} \cdot (\alpha/180)$ (correction)
5. Continuity: forward flow over AV or PV/ VTI_{MV}
   MVA = 0.785 (LVOT D)2 $VTI_{AV}/\ VTI_{MV}$
   Drawbacks: PHT, DT – not as reliable if ASD, PFO, low LV or LA compliance, mod-sev AR – overestimation of MVA (pressure equalizes faster), s/p balloon valvuloplasty

Values for the evaluation of severity of mitral stenosis [7, 8]

	Mild	Moderate	Severe
Area (cm²)	>1.5	1.0–1.5	<1
Mean Gradient (mmHg)- supportive	<5	5–10	>10
PAP (mmHg) – supportive	<30	30–50	>50

Echo score to assess for suitability of mitral balloon valvuloplasty (Wilkins score) [15]

Points	Mobility	Thickening	Calcification	Subvalvular thickening
1	Highly mobile valve with only tips restriction	Leaflets near normal in thickness (4–5 mm)	Single area of increased echo brightness	Minimal thickening just below leaflets
2	Leaflet mid and base portion have normal mobility	Midleaflet normal, considerable thickening of margins (5–8 mm)	Scattered area of brightness confined to leaflet margins	Thickening of chordal structure extending up to 1.3 of chordal length

Points	Mobility	Thickening	Calcification	Subvalvular thickening
3	Valve continues to move forward in diastole mainly from the base	Thickening extends through entire leaflet (5–8 mm)	Brightness extending into midportion of leaflets	Thickening extending to the distal third of chords
4	No or minimal forward movement of leaflets in diastole	Considerable thickening of all leaflet tissue (>8 mm)	Extensive brightness throughout leaflet tissue	Extensive thickening and shortening of all chordal structures extending down to papillary muscles

Score: if <8 – OK to proceed with valvuloplasty, >12 – high risk procedure, consider surgical treatment (Figs. 5.5 and 5.6).

Contraindications to procedure: high score, more than moderate MR, calcific MS, LA thrombus, likely to tear (uneven thickening – will tear where thin), severe TR (procedure does not improve survival (RV failure is already present))

Mitral Regurgitation

Etiologies

Primary (valvular pathology) vs. Secondary (functional from LV or mitral annular dilation)

Primary (Fig. 5.7, Videos 5.7, 5.8, 5.9, and 5.10):

- Myxomatous degeneration with mitral valve prolapse and flail

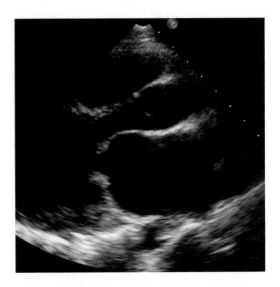

FIGURE 5.5 Low echo score rheumatic mitral stenosis

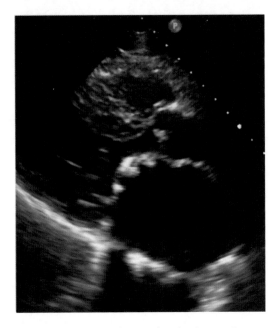

FIGURE 5.6 High echo score rheumatic mitral stenosis

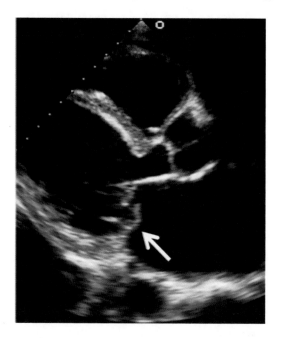

FIGURE 5.7 Flail posterior mitral leaflet (*arrow*); flail occurs when tip of leaflet is in the left atrium

- Endocarditis
- Congenital (cleft mitral valve)
- Rheumatic heart disease

Secondary (Fig. 5.8, Videos 5.11 and 5.12)

- Ischemic and nonischemic cardiomyopathy
- Annular dilation

Evaluation

- – Mitral valve morphology
- – Subvalvular apparatus
- – Left Ventricular size and function
- – Pulmonary Pressures

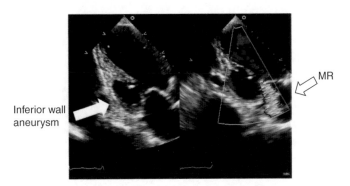

FIGURE 5.8 Ischemic mitral regurgitation. *Left* shows inferior basal aneurysm which has led to apical tethering of the mitral leaflets. This results in restricted closure and severe mitral regurgitation (*right*)

Carpentier classification for Mitral Regurgitation (Based on motion of the mitral leaflets) [16]

Type I: Normal leaf motion. MR due to annular dilatation or leaflet perforation

Type II: Excessive leaflet motion. Prolapse of one or both leaflets due to chordal rupture or elongation

Type III: Restrictive leaflet motion (IIIa Restricted leaflet motion in diastole and systole – leaflet and chordal thickening, commissural fusion due to rheumatic disease, IIIb Restricted leaflet motion during systole – LV enlargement due to ischemic cardiomyopathy)

Useful Formulas

Regurgitant Volume $RV = EROA \cdot VTI_{MR}$

$$RV = \pi / 4 \left(MV\,D\right)^2 \cdot VTI_{MV} - \pi / 4 \left(LVOT\,D\right)^2 \cdot VTI_{LVOT}$$

Regurgitant Fraction $RF = RV / SV = RV / \left(\pi / 4 \left(MV\,D\right)^2 \cdot VTI_{MV}\right)$

EROA $EROA = RV / VTI_{MR}; EROA = 2\pi r^2 \upsilon_{aliasing} / \upsilon_{MR}$

Chronic mitral regurgitation evaluation [8, 13]

	Mild	Moderate	Severe
Color Jet width (cm²)	<4		>8–10
Color jet/LA Area	<20 %		>40 %
Regurgitant Volume (ml)	<30	30–44 mild-mod 45–60 mod-sev	≥60
Regurgitant Fraction	<30 %	30–39 % mild-mod 40–49 mod-sev	≥50
EROA (cm²), Primary MR	<0.2	0.2–0.29 mild-mod 0.3–0.39 mod-sev	≥0.4
EROA (cm²). Secondary MR			≥0.2
Vena Contracta (cm)	<0.3		≥0.7
E			>1.1 m/s (1.2 by some sources)
Mitral inflow	A wave dominant		E wave dominant
MR continuous wave flow	Soft density, parabolic		Dence, triangular
Pulmonary Vein	No or minimal flow convergence		Large flow convergence, systolic reversal

Tricuspid Valve Lesions

Tricuspid Stenosis

Etiology

> Rheumatic heart disease
> Carcinoid syndrome
> Congenital

Evaluation

- Tricuspid valve morphology
- Right Atrial size

Useful formulas

- TVA = 190/PHT
- Right Atrial size

Tricuspid stenosis evaluation [7]

	Severe
Mean Pressure Gradient	≥5 mmHg
Inflow TVI	>60 cm
PHT	≥190 ms
Valve area by continuity equation	≤10 cm^2
RA	≥ moderately enlarged
IVC	Dilated

Tricuspid Regurgitation

Trace or mild degree of TR is present in up to 70 % of normal adults [17].

Etiology

Functional (majority of cases) vs. valvular pathology

Functional:

A. Right atrium, ventricle and tricuspid annulus may dilate due to any condition increasing right ventricular systolic pressure

- Dilated cardiomyopathy
- Left sided heart failure
- Right ventricular infarction
- Mitral stenosis or regurgitation
- Primary pulmonary disease — cor pulmonale, pulmonary hypertension
- Left to right shunts
- Eisenmenger syndrome
- Stenosis of the pulmonic valve or pulmonary artery

B. Tricuspid valve pathology

- infective endocarditis
- valve injury from pacemaker or implantable cardioverter-defibrillator lead placement
- Ebstein's anomaly
- Rheumatic fever
- Carcinoid syndrome
- Connective tissue
- Chest trauma

Evaluation

- Tricuspid valve morphology
- Right Ventricular size and function
- Hepatic Vein
- IVC

Chronic tricuspid regurgitation evaluation [13]

	Mild	Moderate	Severe
Jet area at Nyquist limit (cm^2)	<5	5–10	>10
PISA Radius (cm)	≤0.5	0.6–0.9	>0.9
Jet/RA area (color flow)			>30 %
Regurgitant volume (ml)			>45
EROA (cm^2)			>0.4
Vena Contracta (cm)			>0.7 cm (0.65 cm per echo review)
Tricuspid inflow			>1 m/s
Annular Dilatation			>4 cm
Jet density and contour	Soft, parabolic	Dense, variable	Dense, triangular, early peaking
Hepatic Vein Flow	Systolic dominance	Systolic blunting	Systolic reversal
Tricuspid valve			Abnormal, flail leaflet, poor coaptation
RV/RA/IVC			Dilated

Pulmonary Valve Lesions

Pulmonary Stenosis

Etiology (Subvalvular, Valvular, Supravalvular)

- Congenital (associated with Tetralogy of Fallot, Noonan syndrome, congenital rubella syndrome)
- Carcinoid syndrome

Evaluation

– Pulmonic valve morphology
– Right Ventricular size and function
– Right Ventricular hypertrophy

Pulmonic stenosis evaluation [7]

	Mild	Moderate	Severe
Peak Velocity (m/s)	<3	3–4	>4
Peak Gradient (mmHg)	<36	36–64	>64

Pulmonary Regurgitation

Etiology

– Pulmonary HTN
– Infective endocarditis
– S/p repair of tetralogy of Fallot
– Rheumatic fever

Evaluation

– Pulmonic valve morphology
– Right Ventricular size and function
– Jet size and shape

Pulmonic regurgitation evaluation [13]

	Mild	Moderate	Severe
Jet size by color Doppler	Thin with narrow origin (usually <10 mm in length)		Large, wide origin, may be brief in duration
Jet area/ RVOT area	<25 %	25–50	>50 %

(continued)

	Mild	**Moderate**	**Severe**
Jet density and deceleration rate by CW	Soft, slow deceleration	Dense, variable deceleration time	Dense, steep deceleration, early termination of diastolic flow
Pulmonic systolic flow compared to systemic flow – PW	Slightly increased		Greatly increased
RV size	Normal		Dilated
Pulmonic Valve	Normal		Abnormal

References

1. Roberts WC, Ko JM. Frequency by decades of unicuspid, bicuspid, and tricuspid aortic valves in adults having isolated aortic valve replacement for aortic stenosis, with or without associated aortic regurgitation. Circulation. 2005;111:920–5.
2. Sabet HY, Edwards WD, Tazelaar HD, Daly RV. Congenitally bicuspid aortic valves: a surgical pathology study of 542 cases (1991 through 1996) and a literature review of 2715 additional cases. Mayo Clin Proc. 1999;74:14–26.
3. Siu SC, Silversides CK. Bicuspid aortic valve disease. J Am Coll Cardiol. 2010;55(25):2789–800.
4. Braverman AC, Güven H, Beardslee MA, Makan M, Kates AM, Moon MR. Bicuspid aortic valve. Curr Probl Cardiol. 2005;30: 470–522.
5. Mills P, Leech G, Davies M, Leatham A. The natural history of a non-stenotic bicuspidaortic valve. Br Heart J. 1978;40:951–7.
6. Weyman AE, Scherrer-Crosbie M. Aortic stenosis: physics and physiology – what do the numbers really mean. Rev Cardiovasc Med. 2005;6:23–32.
7. Baumgartner H, Hung J, Bermejo J, Chambers JB, Evangelista A, Griffin BP, Iung B, Otto CM, Pellikka PA, Quiñones M, American Society of Echocardiography; European Association of Echocardiography. Echocardiographic assessment of valve

stenosis: EAE/ASE recommendations for clinical practice. J Am Soc Echocardiogr. 2009;22:1–23.

8. Nishimura RA, Otto CM, Bonow RO, Carabello BA, Erwin 3rd JP, Guyton RA, O'Gara PT, Ruiz CE, Skubas NJ, Sorajja P, Sundt 3rd TM, Thomas JD, ACC/AHA Task Force Members. 2014 AHA/ACC Guideline for the Management of Patients With Valvular Heart Disease: executive summary: a report of the American College of Cardiology/American Heart Association Task Force on Practice Guidelines. Circulation. 2014;129(23):2440–92.

9. Pibarot P, Dumesnil JG. Low-flow, low-gradient aortic stenosis with normal and depressed left ventricular ejection fraction. J Am Coll Cardiol. 2012;60:1845–53.

10. Clavel MA, Fuchs C, Burwash IG, Mundigler G, Dumesnil JG, Baumgartner H, Bergler-Klein J, Beanlands RS, Mathieu P, Magne J, Pibarot P. Predictors of outcomes in low-flow, low-gradient aortic stenosis: results of the multicenter TOPAS Study. Circulation. 2008;118(14 Suppl):S234–42.

11. Monin JL, Quéré JP, Monchi M, Petit H, Baleynaud S, Chauvel C, Pop C, Ohlmann P, Lelguen C, Dehant P, Tribouilloy C, Guéret P. Operative risk stratification and predictors for long-term outcome: a multicenter study using dobutamine stress hemodynamics. Circulation. 2003;108:319–24.

12. Nishimura RA, Grantham JA, Connolly HM, Schaff HV, Higano ST, Holmes DR. Low-output, low-gradient aortic stenosis in patients with depressed left ventricular systolic function. The clinical untility of the dobutamine challenge in the catheterization laboratory. Circulation. 2002;106:809–13.

13. Zoghbi WA, Enriquez-Sarano M, Foster E, Grayburn PA, Kraft CD, Levine RA, Nihoyannopoulos P, Otto CM, Quinones MA, Rakowski H, Stewart WJ, Waggoner A, Weissman NJ, American Society of Echocardiography. Recommendations for evaluation of the severity of native valvular regurgitation with two-dimensional and Doppler echocardiography. J Am Soc Echocardiogr. 2003;16(7):777–802.

14. Tuladhar SM, Punjabi PP. Surgical reconstruction of the mitral valve. Heart. 2006;92:1373–7.

15. Wilkins GT, Weyman AE, Abascal VM, Block PC, Palacios IF. Percutaneous balloon dilatation of the mitral valve: an analysis of echocardiographic variables related to outcome and the mechanism of dilatation. Br Heart J. 1988;60:299–308.

16. Anderson CA, Chitwood WRJR. Advances in mitral valve repair. Future Cardiol. 2009;5:511–6.

17. Lavie CJ, Hebert K, Cassidy M. Prevalence and severity of doppler-detected valvular regurgitation and estimation of right sided cardiac pressures in patients with normal two-dimensional echocardiograms. Chest. 1993;103:226–31.

Chapter 6
Evaluation of Prosthetic Valves

Dmitriy Kireyev and Judy Hung

Abbreviations

AR	Aortic regurgitation
AS	Aortic stenosis
AV	Aortic valve
AVA	Aortic valve area
CO	Cardiac output
EROA	Effective regurgitant orifice area
LVOT	Left ventricular outflow tract
N.B.	Nota bene (lat)
SV	Stroke volume
VTI	Velocity time integral

_____

Electronic supplementary material The online version of this chapter (doi:10.1007/978-3-319-21458-0_6) contains supplementary material, which is available to authorized users.

D. Kireyev, MD (✉) • J. Hung, MD
Echocardiography, Division of Cardiology,
Massachusetts General Hospital, Boston, MA, USA
e-mail: dimonk5@yahoo.com; JHUNG@mgh.harvard.edu

D. Kireyev, J. Hung (eds.), *Cardiac Imaging in Clinical Practice*, In Clinical Practice,
DOI 10.1007/978-3-319-21458-0_6,
© Springer International Publishing Switzerland 2016

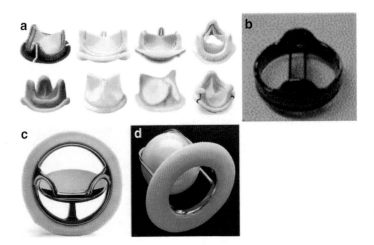

FIGURE 6.1   Shows types of prosthetic valves. (**a**) Bovine pericardial stented valves; (**b**) Mechanical Bileaflet (St Jude Medical Regent, Carbomedics Standard, Medtronic Advantage); (**c**) Single tilting disk (Bjork Shirley, Medtronic-Hall); (**d**) Ball and Cage (Starr-Edwards)

Types of prosthetic valves:

Bioprosthetic: Most common valve is tissue pericardial stented made from bovine pericardium (Fig. 6.1a). Most commonly used mechanical valves are Bileaflet tilting disc (St Jude Medical Regent, Carbomedics Standard, Medtronic Advantage Fig. 6.1b), Single tilting disk (Bjork Shirley, Medtronic-Hall) (Fig. 6.1c) and Ball and Cage type valves (Starr-Edwards) are no longer used (Fig. 6.1d).

The first valve implantation was performed by Charles Hufnagel in 1952.

Hufnagel CA, Harvey WP, Rabil PJ, McDermott TM. Surgical correction of aortic insufficiency. *Surgery* 1954,35:673–83

Prosthetic Valves

Aortic Prosthesis Stenosis

Parameter	Normal	Possible stenosis	Significant stenosis
Peak V(m/s)	<3	3–4	>4
Mean gradient (mmHg)	<20	20–35	>35
DVI (V_{LVOT}/V_{PrV} vs VTIs)	≥0.3	0.25–0.29	<0.25
ERO (cm²)	>1.2	0.8–1.2	<0.8
Contour of jet velocity	Triangular, early peaking	Triangular to semi rounded	Rounded, symmetrical
Acceleration time (ms) [2]	<80	80–100	>100

Videos 6.1 and 6.2 show images of a 12 year old aortic bioprosthesis. The prosthetic aortic leaflets are significantly thickened and calcified and color Doppler flow shows turbulent flow across prosthesis consistent elevated gradients (Fig. 6.2). Figure 6.3 shows spectral Doppler profile of elevated peak gradient of 80 mmHg with an acceleration time of 160 ms across a bioprosthetic aortic valve consistent with significant prosthetic valve stenosis.

Aortic Prosthesis Regurgitation

Parameter	Mild	Moderate	Severe
Valve structure	Nl	Abnormal	Abnormal
LV size	Nl		Enlarged
Jet width/LVOT diameter	≤25 %	26–64 %	≥65
Jet density	Faint		Dense
Jett deceleration PHT (ms)	>500	200–500	<200

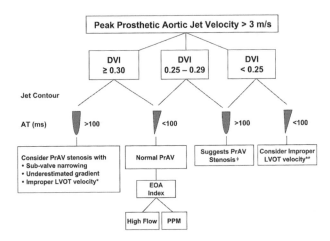

FIGURE 6.2 Algorithm of assessment of peak prosthetic aortic jet velocity >3 m/s (Reproduced with permission from Zoghbi et al. [1]. *, ** - PW sample located too close and too far from the valve, respectively. φ compare derived EOA to the reference values for the valve for further analysis. http://dx.doi.org/10.1016/j.echo.2009.07.013. © 2009 American Society of Echocardiography. Published by Elsevier Inc)

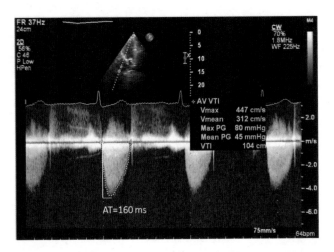

FIGURE 6.3 shows elevated peak gradient of 80 mmHg with an acceleration time of 160 ms across a bioprosthetic aortic valve consistent with significant prosthetic valve stenosis

Parameter	Mild	Moderate	Severe
LVOT flow vs. pulmonic flow (PW)	Slightly increased		Greatly increased
Diastolic reversal in descending aorta	Absent or early diastolic		Prominent holodiastolic
Regurgitant volume (ml/bt)	<30	30–59	>60
Regurgitant fraction	<30	30–50	>50

Example of a paravalvular aortic prosthetic valve regurgitation as seen on 3D transesophageal imaging is demonstrated in Video 6.3.

Patient prosthesis mismatch: EOAindex = Stroke Volume/ $(VTI_{PrV} \times BSA)$

EOA >**0.85 cm²/m²** not significant; EOA **0.65–0.85 cm²/m²** moderate; EOA <**0.65 cm²** severe

Prosthetic Mitral Valve Stenosis

Parameter	Normal	Possible stenosis	Significant stenosis
Peak velocity (m/s)	<1.9	1.9–2.5	≥2.5
Mean gradient (mmHg)	≤5	5–10	>10
DVI (VTI_{PrV}/VTI_{LVOT})	<2.2	2.2–2.5	>2.5
ERO (cm²)	≥2	1–2	<1
PHT(ms)	<130	130–200	>200

Video 6.4 shows a patient with St. Jude mitral prosthesis with prolonged subtherapeutic INR. Video shows a stuck prosthetic disc resulting in significant mitral stenosis.

Prosthetic Mitral Valve Regurgitation (TEE + TTE)

Parameter	Mild	Moderate	Severe
LV size			Enlarge
Prosthetic valve morphology			Abnormal
Color flow jet area (Niquist 50–60 cm/s)	Small central (<4 cm), <20 %		>8 cm^2, >40 %
Flow convergence			Large
Jet density			Dense
Jet contour	Parabolic		Early peaking triangular
Pulmonic vein flow	Systolic dominance		Systolic flow reversal
Vena contracta (cm^2)	<0.3		≥0.6
Regurgitant Volume (ml/beat)	<30		≥60
Regurgitant fraction	<30		≥50
EROA (cm^2)	<0.2		≥0.5

Examples of paravalvular mitral prosthetic valve regurgitation are demonstrated in Videos 6.5 and 6.6.

Examples of paravalvular mitral prosthetic valve regurgitation is demonstrated in Videos 6.4 and 6.4.

Interesting fact: the first intracardiac mechanical valve prosthesis: Starr Edward valve was implanted in a patient with severe mitral regurgitation and stage IV heart failure on 8/25/1960 (Starr A, Edwards ML. Mitral replacement: clinical experience with a ball-valve prosthesis. *Annals of Surgery* 1961;154:726–40)

Prosthetic Tricuspid Stenosis

Average data over 5 cycles
Suspicion for severe stenosis:

Peak velocity (m/s)	>1.7
Mean gradient (mmHg)	≥6
PHT (ms)	≥230

Prosthetic Tricuspid Valve Regurgitation

Parameter	Mild	Moderate	Severe
Valve structure	normal		Abnormal, valve dehiscence
Jet area by Doppler (central jet only)	<5	5–10	>10
Vena Contracta (cm)	Not defined		>0.7
Jet density and contour by CW	faint		Dense, early peaking
Doppler systolic hepatic flow	Normal or blunter		Holosystolic reversal
RA, RV, IVC			

Prosthetic Pulmonic Valve Stenosis

Suspect stenosis if:

• Peak velocity >3 m/s (or >2 m/s for homograph)
• Abnormal morphology
• Impaired RV, increased RVSP

Prosthetic Pulmonic Regurgitation

Parameter	Mild	Severe
Jet size/pulmonary annulus by Doppler (central jet)	<25 %	>50 %
Jet density (CW)		Dense
Jet deceleration (CW)		Slow
Pulmonic systolic flow vs. systemic flow		Greatly increased
Diastolic flow reversal Pulmonary artery		Present
RV		Enlarged
Valve structure		Abnormal

Prosthetic Valve Complications

Common prosthetic valve complications are:

Prosthetic valve endocarditis with vegetation (Fig. 6.4; Video 6.7)
Prosthetic valve abscess (Figs. 6.5 and 6.6).
Prosthetic valve dehiscence (Video 6.8)
Prosthetic valve abscess with fistula (Video 6.9)

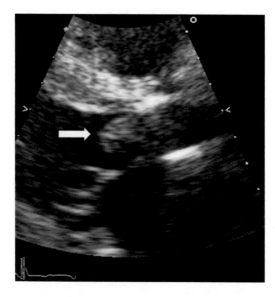

FIGURE 6.4 Transthoracic parasternal image of a large prosthetic aortic valve vegetation in the LVOT (*arrow*)

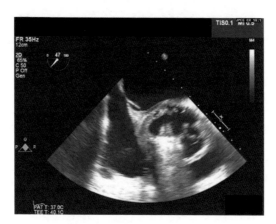

FIGURE 6.5 Transesophageal image of short axis of aortic root abscess in patient with prosthetic valve endocarditis. Note thickening with irregular echodensities of the aortic sinuses

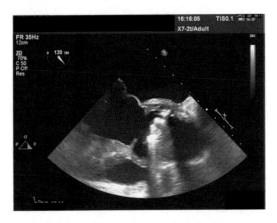

FIGURE 6.6 Transesophageal image of long axis of aorta in patient with prosthetic valve endocarditis and aortic root abscess. Note thickening with irregular echodensities of the aortic sinuses

References

1. Zoghbi WA, Chambers JB, Dumesnil JG, Foster E, Gottdiener JS, Grayburn PA, Khandheria BK, Levine RA, Marx GR, Miller Jr FA, Nakatani S, Quiñones MA, Rakowski H, Rodriguez LL, Swaminathan M, Waggoner AD, Weissman NJ, Zabalgoitia M, American Society of Echocardiography's Guidelines and Standards Committee; Task Force on Prosthetic Valves; American College of Cardiology Cardiovascular Imaging Committee; Cardiac Imaging Committee of the American Heart Association; European Association of Echocardiography; European Society of Cardiology; Japanese Society of Echocardiography; Canadian Society of Echocardiography; American College of Cardiology Foundation; American Heart Association; European Association of Echocardiography; European Society of Cardiology; Japanese Society of Echocardiography; Canadian Society of Echocardiography. Recommendations for evaluation of prosthetic valves with echocardiography and Doppler ultrasound: a report From the American Society of Echocardiography's Guidelines and Standards Committee and the Task Force on Prosthetic Valves, developed in conjunction with the American College of Cardiology Cardiovascular Imaging Committee,

Cardiac Imaging Committee of the American Heart Association, the European Association of Echocardiography, a registered branch of the European Society of Cardiology, the Japanese Society of Echocardiography and the Canadian Society of Echocardiography, endorsed by the American College of Cardiology Foundation, American Heart Association, European Association of Echocardiography, a registered branch of the European Society of Cardiology, the Japanese Society of Echocardiography, and Canadian Society of Echocardiography. J Am Soc Echocardiogr. 2009;22(9):975–1014.

2. Ben Zekry S, Saad RM, Ozkan M, Al Shahid MS, Pepi M, Muratori M, Xu J, Little SH, Zoghbi WA. Flow acceleration time and ratio of acceleration time to ejection time for prosthetic aortic valve function. JACC Cardiovasc Imaging. 2011;4(11):1161–70.

Chapter 7
Diastolic Function

Dmitriy Kireyev and Judy Hung

Diastolic dysfunction (impaired left ventricular relaxation) is found in a significant proportion of patients presenting with heart failure. It is found in both patients with preserved (Heart Failure with preserved Ejection Fraction (HFpEF)) and decreased systolic heart function (Heart Failure with reduced Ejection Fraction (HFrEF)). Diastolic dysfunction leads to the elevated filling pressures which subsequently may cause congestive symptoms and left atrial changes.

Echocardiography helps to both assess the impaired left ventricular relaxation as well as its consequences.

Echocardiographic assessment of LV diastolic dysfunction.

D. Kireyev, MD (✉) • J. Hung, MD
Echocardiography, Division of Cardiology,
Massachusetts General Hospital, Boston, MA, USA
e-mail: dimonk5@yahoo.com; JHUNG@mgh.harvard.edu

D. Kireyev, J. Hung (eds.), *Cardiac Imaging in Clinical Practice*, In Clinical Practice,
DOI 10.1007/978-3-319-21458-0_7,
© Springer International Publishing Switzerland 2016

LV Chambers

- Assess left ventricle for hypertrophy (both concentric and eccentric). Assess left ventricular function – patients with left ventricular dysfunction also have impaired relaxation
- Assess LV geometry
- Assess interventricular interactions
- Assess left atrial size (volume) and volume index (Note: normal heart adaptation in athletes, cardiomyopathies, mitral stenosis, atrial fibrillation, shunts and high output states may increase left atrial size in the absence of diastolic dysfunction).
- Assess pulmonary artery pressure (note: can be elevated due to pulmonary disease, etc.)

Mitral Inflow Patterns

- Acquire Pulse Wave Doppler mitral inflow profile from apical 4 chamber view placing a sample volume between mitral leaflet tips. Pulse wave Doppler should be used, (also Continuous wave Doppler should be used to double check peak E (early diastolic filling) and A (late diastolic filling) wave velocities).
- Measure: E, A, E/A, deceleration time (DT), IVRT (isovolumic relaxation time), A wave duration (obtain at the Mitral annulus level)

  E wave determinants: pressure gradient between LA and LV during early diastole, LA compliance, LV elastic recoil,

  A wave determinants: pressure gradient between LA and LV during late diastole, LV compliance, LA contractile function

  E wave deceleration time (DT) determinants: LV compliance, relaxation, diastolic pressures,

N.B. In patients with CAD or HCM with EF ≥50 % mitral valve parameters correlated poorly with hemodynamic parameters [1–3].

N.B.2 E/A ratio is often <1 in normal subjects above the age of 60 [1].

Tissue Doppler

- Use Pulse Wave Tissue Doppler to acquire mitral annular velocities from apical views positioning sample volume within 1 cm of septal and lateral insertion sites. Measurements should be done at end-expiration.
- Obtain S (systolic velocity), e′ (early diastolic velocity) and a′ (late diastolic velocity)

e′ determinants: LV relaxation, LV function and preload.

A′ determinant: LVEDP and LA contractile function.

E/e′ is used to predict LV filling pressures (<8 is seen in patients with normal and >15 with elevated filing pressures)

N.B. e′ septal is usually lower than e′ lateral

Limitations: patients with MAC, mitral rings, mitral stenosis, prosthetic mitral valves.

Pulmonary Venous Flow

- Acquire Pulse Wave Doppler of pulmonary venous flow in the apical 4 chamber view placing a sample volume more than 5 mm into pulmonary vein.
- Measure S (systolic velocity; use S2 since S1 is related to atrial relaxation), D (peak anterograde diastolic velocity), S2/D ratio, Ar (peak velocity in late diastole), Ar duration

N.B. Duration of A_{mitral} – Duration of $A_{pulmonic}$ >30 ms indicated elevated LVEDP [1].

Color M-Mode Propagation Velocity

- Measures mitral to apical flow propagation
- Use apical 4 chamber view, place M-mode scan line in the center on LV inflow blood stream from mitral valve to the apex, use color flow imaging. Decrease Nyquist limit to have the central jet in blue.
- Flow propagation velocity is a slope of the first aliasing velocity during early filling measured 4 cm into the LV cavity.
- Propagation velocity of <50 cm/s is abnormal

Valsalva Maneuver Use for Distinguishing Normal Versus Pseudo Normal Patterns of Relaxation

Pseudo normal mitral inflow pattern is sometimes hard to distinguish from the normal pattern creating a potential for test misinterpretation.

Valsalva maneuver decreases the preload (stage II, strain stage)

In normal subjects both E and A decrease proportionally and thus E/A ration is not significantly changed. In subjects with pseudo normal pattern E and A velocities decrease at different rates and E/A ration is moved to impaired relaxation range.

N.B. a decrease of E velocity by 20 cm/s shows that Valsalva maneuver was adequate.

N.B.2 In the absence of adequate Valsalva maneuver, assess tissue Doppler e′ and e′/a′ ratio – it would be abnormal in pseudo normal diastolic pattern

Diastolic Dysfunction

	DT (ms)	E/A	E/E′	E′ (cm)	IVRT (ms)	P$_{vs2}$ P$_{vp}$	Mitral A vs PulmA
Normal	160–240	>1.5	<8	10	–	–	–
I	>240	<1	≤8 (1a >15)	–	>90	∧	Depend on LVEDD
II	160–220	1–1.5	>15 lateral wall >12 septal wall	<7	<90	∨	∨
III/IV	<160	>1.5	>15 lateral wall >12 septal wall	<7	<70	∨∨	∨

Caveats:

- Data in elderly and pediatric population is not well validated
- Grading correlation is not absolute

Figure 7.1 shows an example of high E/E′ ratio consistent with elevated LV filling pressures. Recommendations on evaluation of diastolic function and left atrial pressure can also be found at the following link: (http://www.onlinejase. com/article/S0894-7317(08)00739-6/fulltext).

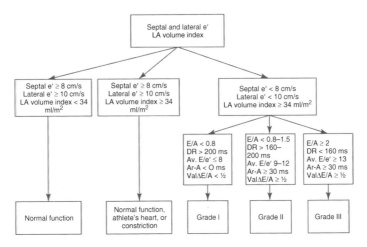

FIGURE 7.1 Diagnostic algorithm for evaluation of diastolic disfunction severity [1]

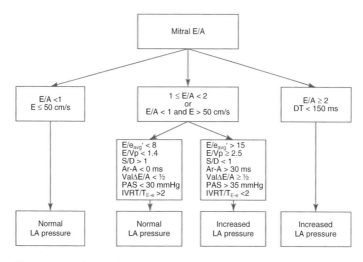

FIGURE 7.2 Diagnostic algorithm for evaluation of filling pressures in patient with normal Ejection fraction [1]

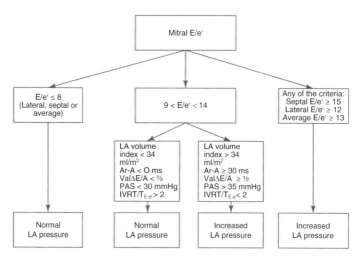

FIGURE 7.3 Diagnostic algorithm for evaluation of filling pressures in patient with lowered Ejection fraction [1]

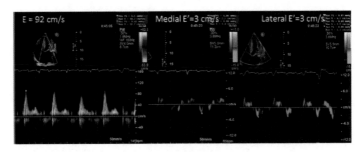

FIGURE 7.4 Pulse and tissue Doppler imaging showing an example of high E/E′ ratio consistent with elevated LV filling pressures

Reference

1. Nagueh SF, Appleton CP, Gillebert TC, Marino PN, Oh JK, Smiseth OA, Waggoner AD, Flachskampf FA, Pellikka PA, Evangelista A. Recommendations for the evaluation of left ventricular diastolic function by echocardiography. J Am Soc Echocardiogr. 2009;22(2):107–33.
2. Nagueh SF, Lakkis NM, Middleton KJ, Spencer WHIII, Zoghbi WA, Quinones MA. Doppler estimation of left ventricular filling pressures in patients with hypertrophic cardiomyopathies. Circulation 1999;99:254–61.
3. Nishimura RA, Appleton CP, Redfield MM, Ilstrup DM, Holmes DR Jr, Tajik AJ. Noninvasive Doppler echocardiographic evaluation of left ventricular filling pressures in patients with cardiomyopathies: a simultaneous Doppler echocardiographic and cardiac catheterization study. J Am Coll Cardiol 1997;30:1819–26.

Chapter 8
Pericardial Disease

Dmitriy Kireyev and Judy Hung

Echocardiography is a portable and readily available technique for the evaluation of pericardial disease. Pericardial thickening (Fig. 8.1), effusion, masses, constrictions, effusive-constrictive pericarditis, congenital absence of pericardium are some of the conditions which may be evaluated from both anatomical and hemodynamic perspectives.

Electronic supplementary material The online version of this chapter (doi:10.1007/978-3-319-21458-0_8) contains supplementary material, which is available to authorized users.

D. Kireyev, MD (✉) • J. Hung, MD
Echocardiography, Division of Cardiology,
Massachusetts General Hospital, Boston, MA, USA
e-mail: dimonk5@yahoo.com; JHUNG@mgh.harvard.edu

D. Kireyev, J. Hung (eds.), *Cardiac Imaging in Clinical Practice*, In Clinical Practice,
DOI 10.1007/978-3-319-21458-0_8,
© Springer International Publishing Switzerland 2016

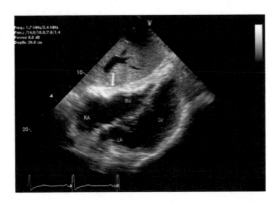

FIGURE 8.1 Subcostal view showing heart with significant pericardial thickening (*arrow*)

Pericardial Effusion (Fig. 8.1)

Determine:

- Size (Size criteria differ between publications). Measure in diastole: trivial 1–5 mm, small 5 mm-1 cm, moderate 1–3 cm, large >3 cm
- Circumferential vs. loculated (Loculated effusions are more common after surgery, trauma, purulent pericarditis)
- Fluid characteristics: look for fibrin strands, echogenic masses

Assess for cardiac tamponade (Figs. 8.2, 8.3, 8.4, and 8.5, Videos 8.1 and 8.2)

- Exaggerated respiratory variations in mitral and tricuspid inflow profiles. Cut offs 30 % MV, 60 % TV [1]
- Right atrium inversion (greater than 1/3 of cardiac cycle)
- Right ventricular diastolic inversion
- IVC dilatation and reduced respiratory changes in diameter (<50 % decrease)

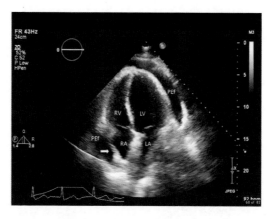

FIGURE 8.2 Apical 4 chamber view showing circumferential pericardial effusion (*PEf*). The *arrow* shows right atrial collapse during late diastole

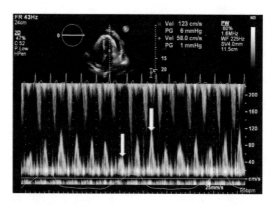

FIGURE 8.3 Doppler mitral valve flow profile in patient with pericardial effusion. Note the variability of mitral valve inflow pattern (*arrows*) during the respiratory cycle (*green curve* on the bottom of the image represents patients breathing pattern). Significant increase of mitral flow with expiration and decrease with inspiration suggests tamponade physiology

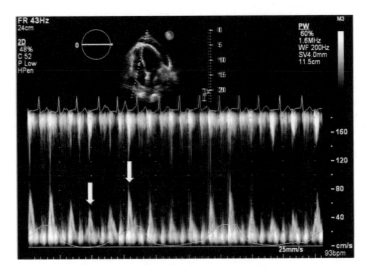

FIGURE 8.4 Doppler tricuspid valve flow profiles in patient with pericardial effusion (*arrows*). Note the significant increase in inflow during the inspiration and decrease with expiration suggesting tamponade physiology

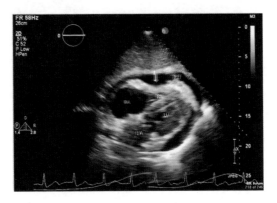

FIGURE 8.5 Subxyphoid view of pericardial effusion (*PEf*). Note the early diastolic right ventricular collapse (*arrow*) consistent with tamponade physiology

Pericardial Cysts (Fig. 8.6)

- Rare
- Most are asymptomatic
- May look like localized pericardial effusion
- May be either multilocular

Constrictive Pericarditis

- Consider the diagnosis in patients with ascites, chronic venous congestion, elevated jugular venous pressure, peripheral edema
- Often caused by chronic inflammation of pericardium
- Thickened pericardium is not obligatory
- Pericardium constraint causes interventricular dependence (with inspiration increased filling of right ventricle causes interventricular septum (IVS) to move left and with expiration the increased filling of left ventricle causes IVC to move left)

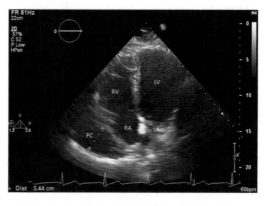

FIGURE 8.6 Apical four chamber view showing pericardial cyst (*PC*) located adjacent to the right atrium

- Paradoxical motion if IVS (during atrial filling exaggerated anterior movement of IVS, during the early diastole posterior movement of the IVS as right ventricle fills prior to left one)
- Increased ventricular filling during early diastole due to elevated atrial pressures
- Exaggerated inflow changes with respiratory cycle
- IVC dilatation and reduced respiratory changes in diameter (<50 % decrease)

Constrictive Pericarditis Versus Restrictive Cardiomyopathy by Echo

Constriction is more likely when:

- Relaxation parameters are not affected
- Exaggerated respiratory MV and TV flow variation
- Normal tissue Doppler velocities
- E ≥8 cm/s (90 % sensitive, 100 % specific) [2]
- Slope of ≥100 cm/s for the first aliasing slope by color M-mode (74 % sensitive, 91 % specific) [1]
- Increased respiratory variation in pulmonary D wave
- Pulmonary S and D waves are approximately equal in size (D >>> S in restriction)
- Septal bounce with respiration is present
- Presence of diastolic mitral regurgitation

Congenital Absence of Pericardium

- Rare
- May be partial or complete
- Variable clinical presentation. The most common concern is herniation of the part of the heart leading to hemodynamic changes [3]

- Frequently picked up incidentally in CXR (heart malposition)
- Features

  unusual echocardiographic windows
  cardiac hypermobility
  abnormal ventricular septal motion
  abnormal swinging motion of the heart in seven patients.

References

1. Klein AL, Abbara S, Agler DA, Appleton CP, Asher CR, Hoit B, Hung J, Garcia MJ, Kronzon I, Oh JK, Rodriguez ER, Schaff HV, Schoenhagen P, Tan CD, White RD. American Society of Echocardiography clinical recommendations for multimodality cardiovascular imaging of patients with pericardial disease: endorsed by the Society for Cardiovascular Magnetic Resonance and Society of Cardiovascular Computed Tomography. J Am Soc Echocardiogr. 2013;26(9):965–1012.
2. Rajagopalan N, Garcia MJ, Rodriguez L, Murray RD, Apperson-Hansen C, Stugaard M, Thomas JD, Klein AL. Comparison of new Doppler echocardiographic methods to differentiate constrictive pericardial heart disease and restrictive cardiomyopathy. Am J Cardiol. 2001;87(1):86–94.
3. Connolly HM, Click RL, Schattenberg TT, Seward JB, Tajik AJ. Congenital absence of the pericardium: echocardiography as a diagnostic tool. J Am Soc Echocardiogr. 1995;8(1):87–92.

Chapter 9
Cardiac Masses

Dmitriy Kireyev and Judy Hung

Cardiac Tumors

Primary vs. Secondary
Benign vs. Malignant

Interesting fact: cardiac tumor was first described by an Italian professor of anatomy and surgeon at University of Padua Matteo Realdo Colombo (alternatively Matteo Renaldus Columbus) in 1559 [1]. He is also famous for proposing pulmonary circulation and discovering that the primary function of the heart is contraction.

Electronic supplementary material The online version of this chapter (doi:10.1007/978-3-319-21458-0_9) contains supplementary material, which is available to authorized users.

D. Kireyev, MD (✉) • J. Hung, MD
Echocardiography, Division of Cardiology,
Massachusetts General Hospital, Boston, MA, USA
e-mail: dimonk5@yahoo.com; JHUNG@mgh.harvard.edu

D. Kireyev, J. Hung (eds.), *Cardiac Imaging in Clinical Practice*, In Clinical Practice,
DOI 10.1007/978-3-319-21458-0_9,
© Springer International Publishing Switzerland 2016

Secondary Tumors in the Heart (Fig. 9.1)

Significantly more common than primary tumors. The tumors get in the heart via bloodstream, lymphatics, direct extension and extension via vena cava or pulmonary veins.

Leukemias, melanomas, thyroid carcinomas, lung cancers, sarcomas, esophageal cancer, renal cell cancer, lymphomas, breast cancer and malignant mesotheliomas are some of the more common primary cancers [2].

Primary Cardiac Tumors

- Extremely rare (<0.056 % per review of 12,485 autopsies by Lam et al.; 0.0017 % per review of 480,331 cases by Straus and Merlis) [3, 4]

Benign Tumors

Myxoma (Fig. 9.2, Video 9.1)

Most common primary cardiac tumors, up to 50 % of surgically resected primary cardiac tumors [5].

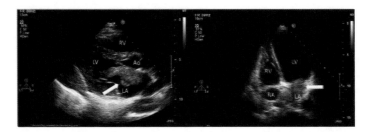

FIGURE 9.1 Parasternal long axis (*left*) and apical four chamber (*right*) views showing epithelial lung tumor extension (*arrows*) in the left atrium. CT reconstruction showed direct extension of the tumor from right pulmonary vein into the left atrium

Women more commonly affected than man.

More frequently appear between 3rd and 6th decade of life.

Morphology

often pedunculated. Surface is smooth, friable or villous. Internally may contain cysts and areas of necrosis and hemorrhage.

Location

75 % – left atrium, 20 % – right atrium [6]. Tumors often arise at the interatrial septum at the border of fossa ovalis membrane [7].

Symptoms

emboli; symptoms of mitral valve obstruction, fever, weight loss, anemia, elevated CRP [8].

Associations

Carney complex – Autosomal Dominant; multiple tumors – myxomas (presenting earlier, sometimes multiple, more likely to recur), schwannomas, endocrine tumours, blue nevi, pigmented lentigines

LAMB – **l**entigines, **a**trial myxomas, **m**ucocutaneous myxomas, **b**lue nevi

NAME – **n**evi, **a**trial myxomas, **m**yxoid neurofibomas, **e**phelides

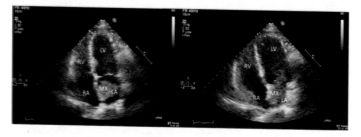

FIGURE 9.2 Apical four chamber view showing left atrial myxoma (*MX*) in systole (*left*) and diastole (*right*). Note the myxoma prolapsing through the mitral valve causing the obstruction

Imaging

> Echo: Evaluate location, size, mobility, possible valvular obstruction
>
> CT or MRI (increased intensity on T2 weighted images) – usually not needed. May help with location of attachment if not readily seen by echo.

Treatment

> surgical resection

Recurrence [5, 8]

> Sporadic tumors – 3 %
> Familial mycomas – 22 %
> Recurrence frequency increases linearly for up to 4 years after which it decreases significantly
> Site of recurrence is the same as original location of tumor in 81 % of cases
> Follow up semiannually for 4 years after resection

Papillary Fibroelastoma (Fig. 9.3, Video 9.2)

Second most common primary cardiac tumors [9].
> Men are more commonly affected.

Morphology

Pedunculated, highly papillary, avascular tumour covered by a layer of endothelium. Tumors resemble sea anemones when placed in normal saline.

Location

Most originate from the valves:
Aortic > Mitral > Tricuspid > Pulmonic.
Ninety-five percent in the left side of the heart [9].

Symptoms

Most patients are asymptomatic. Presentation may involve embolic events from both tumors (partial or whole) and thrombi attached to it (strokes, TIA, visual loss, angina, infarction, syncope, death), aortic or pulmonic stenosis symptoms.

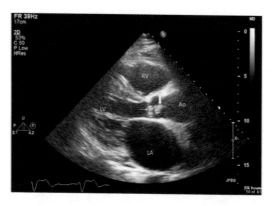

FIGURE 9.3 Parasternal long axis view showing Papillary Fibroelastoma (*thick arrow*) attached to the aortic valve (*thin arrow*)

Imaging

Echo: small, mobile mass which is often pedunculated. Central echolucency may be present. Tumors often appear speckled and have stippled pattern near the edges ("shimmering edge")
CT and MRI – usually not necessary.

Treatment

large (≥1 cm) mobile and symptomatic tumours usually are resected [8, 9]. Some specialists recommend resection of tumors given potentially devastating consequenced of embolization. Consider observation and possible antiplatelet/anticoagulation therapy for others. Surgery is curative.

Lipoma (Fig. 9.4)

Morphology

Accumulation of adipocytes

Location

50 % subendocardial origin
More frequently located in the ventricles

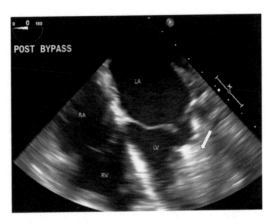

FIGURE 9.4 Transesophageal four chamber view showing massive cardiac lipoma (*arrow*) in the left ventricle which is extending into the mitral valve

Symptoms

usually asymptomatic
If present, are due to arrhythmias, heart block, compression of coronary arteries

Imaging

Echo: helps with size and location

CT and MRI – may be useful for diagnosis since lipomas have distinctive fat imaging pattern
Treatment

surgery if symptomatic

N.B. Lipomatous septal hypertrophy is not a tumor, but rather a benign hyperplasia of adipose tissues in the limbus of the fossa ovalis. Since thin part of interatrial septum (fosssa ovalis) is not involved, a typical "dumbell shaped" image is seen on 2D echo

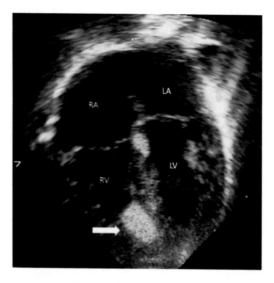

FIGURE 9.5 Echocardiogram (note the different orientation) showing right ventricular rhabdomyoma (*arrow*); orientation is inverted with atria on top and ventricles on bottom

Rhabdomyoma (Fig. 9.5)

Most common primary cardiac neoplasm in children [10].

Morphology

Microscopically consist of "spider cells" – striated cells with features of myocytes.

Tumor cells loose the ability to divide and may regress spontaneously in both size and number [1, 8, 11].

Location

Tumors are usually multiple and located in ventricles [6].

Symptoms

arrhythmias, heart block, flow obstruction

Associations

Very strong association with tuberous sclerosis, ventricular pre-excitation and Wolff-Parkinson-White syndrome [8].

Imaging

> Echocardiography: round, usually well delineated echogenic masses which have a slightly higher intensity than surrounding myocardium [8,12]. Echocardiography helps to evaluate location, size and significance of obstruction, if any.
>
> CT – hypodense masses on contrast CT
>
> MRI – T1 weighted images – isointense, T2 weighted images – hyperintense. MRI is useful for differentiation of rhabdomyoma from fibroma which is also common in children [3, 13].

Treatment

observation (since there is often a spontaneous remission) and surgery in symptomatic patients

Fibroma (Fig. 9.6)

Second most common benign tumor in children and most common resected cardiac tumor in children [14].

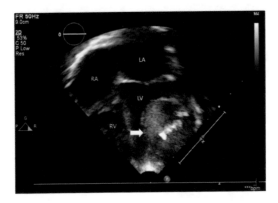

FIGURE 9.6 Large fibroma (*arrow*) with areas of calcification in the left atrium. orientation is inverted with atria on top and ventricles on bottom

Morphology

consists of fibroblasts interspersed among collagen. Occasional calcifications and ossification foci are noted [6, 8].

Location

> Usually ventricular septum and left ventricular free wall [14].
> Tumor is usually solitary

Associations

Gorlin syndrome (also known as Gorlin Goltz syndrome and nevoid basal cell carcinoma syndrome (NBCCS))): Autosomal dominant condition associated with: multiple and early onset basal cell carcinomas, recurrent odontogenic cysts in the jaw, pits on palms and soles, rib anomalies, calcified falx cerebri, cardiac fibromas, melanomas, ovarian fibromas and other tumors [15].

Symptoms

arrhythmias, heart blocks, heart failure, outflow obstruction, sudden death

Imaging

> Echocardiography: echogenic solid non-contractile mass.
> CT: homogeneous mass with soft tissue attenuation with possible foci of calcification [13].
> MRI: T2 images: homogeneous and hypointense masses. T1: isointense relative to myocardium [13]. Little or no contrast enhancement.

Treatment

Surgery in symptomatic patients. Consider surgery in asymptomatic patients due to high risk of sudden cardiac death.

Malignant Tumors

15–25 % of primary cardiac tumors are malignant [8, 10].

Sarcomas (Fig. 9.7, Video 9.3)

More than 90 % of malignant cardiac tumors are sarcomas [5].

Morphology

histologic types: angiosarcomas, rhabdosarcomas, leiomyo-sarcomas, fibrosarcomas, liposarcomas, osteosarcmoas, synovial sarcomas and undifferentiated sarcomas (note: it is not clear if histologic subtype affects prognosis)

Location

> Angiosarcomas (most common) more common in the right atrium or pericardium
>
> Rhabdomyosarcomas (second most common) – extensive myocardial infiltration
>
> Leiomyosarcomas – more common in left atrium
>
> Metastasis: extensions are often epicardial, endocardial, intracavitary pleaural, pulmonary venous, etc.

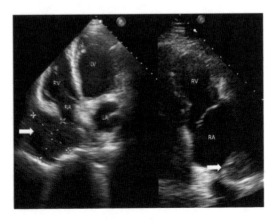

FIGURE 9.7 Four chamber (*left image*) and RV inflow (*right image*) view of patient with right atrial angiosarcoma (*arrows*)

Symptoms often non-specific, systemic (fever, weight loss), dyspnea, palpitations, arrhythmias, conduction defects, congestive heart failure, obstruction, embolism.

Note: 80 % of sarcomas already have metastasis at the point of diagnosis [6].

Imaging

Echocardiography: possible presentation: angiosarcomas – right atrial mass, leiomyosarcomas – left atrial mass, osteosarcomas – may be seen near the junction of pulmonary veins (TEE may be preferred to TTE)

CT, MRI – permit definitive diagnosis, especially for angiosarcoma which shows arterial phase inhancement.

Treatment

Poor prognosis, median survival of 1 year

Roles of chemotherapy, radiation therapy, surgical resection and cardiac transplantation are controversial due to lack of data.

Primary Cardiac Lymphoma, Mesotheliomas, Plasmocytomas, and Paragangliomas Are Extremely Rare

Other Masses Encountered in the Heart

Lambl's Excrescences (Fig. 9.8)

Interesting fact: Lambl's excrescences were first described by Vilém Dušan Lambl in 1856 [16].

Morphology

filiform or lamellar [17]. Consist of core of connective tissue covered by endothelium.

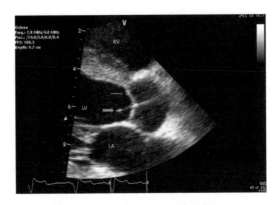

FIGURE 9.8 Enlarged parasternal long axis view showing Lambl's excrescence (*thick arrow*) attached to the aortic valve (*thin arrow*)

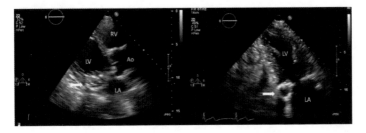

FIGURE 9.9 Parasternal long axis (left) and apical 2 chamber (*right*) views showing caseous calcification of posterior annulus of the mitral valve (*arrow*)

Location

often observed on aortic and mitral valves.

Symptoms

may present with embolic events.

Caseous Calcification of the Mitral Annulus (Liquification Necrosis of Mitral Annulus) (Fig. 9.9)

   Chronic degenerative process with involvement of posterior annulus (in most cases).
   Variant of mitral annular calcification

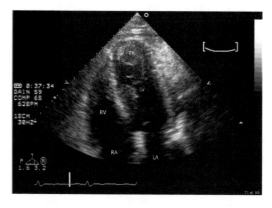

FIGURE 9.10 Apical four chamber view showing LV thrombus (*Th*)

more common in elderly and women (0.64–2.7 % of patients with MAC) [18, 19].
mixture of calcium, fatty acids and cholesterol

Imaging

Echocardiography: round, echo dense mass with smooth borders may contain areas of echo lucency
CT: hyperdense mass with calcified edges
MRI: mass with hyperintense central area and hypointense rim on T1 weighted fast spin echo or T 1 weighted spoiled gradient echo [20].
Prognosis: Usually benign

Intracardiac Thrombi (Figs. 9.10, 9.11, 9.12, and 9.13, Videos 9.4, 9.5, and 9.6)

Appear as a result of conditions predisposing to hemostasis and stagnant blood flow.

Spontaneous echocardiographic contrast (smoke) is a sign of stagnant flow and is considered a predisposition of thrombus formation.

Location

Ventricular

Associated with myocardial infarction, myocarditis, cardiomyopathy or aneurysm (Fig. 9.10)
Associated with left ventricular non-compaction

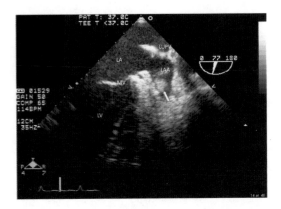

FIGURE 9.11 Transesophageal echocardiogram showing left atrial appendage thrombus (*arrow*). Left upper pulmonary vein (*LUPV*) can be seen in this view

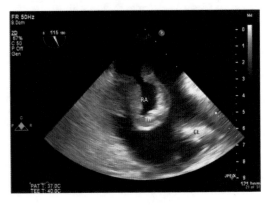

FIGURE 9.12 Modified bicaval view, Transesophageal echocardiogram. Notice large right atrial thrombus (*Th*). CL – Central Line Catheter

Atrial

Atrial fibrillation and left atrial appendage thrombus due to stagnant flow (thrombus +/− low LAA velocity image)

Prosthetic valve or intra-cardiac devices (including pacemakers, defibrillators and central lines)

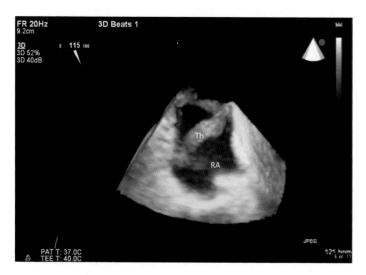

FIGURE 9.13 A 3D reconstruction of the thrombus in the left atrium (From Figure 9.8.3)

Thrombus formation on top of papillary fibroelastoma or myxoma

Symptoms

due to embolization or obstruction

Treatment

reversal/removal of underlying etiology, anticoagulation, thrombectomy (Vortex or surgical)

Vegetations (Figs. 9.14, 9.15, 9.16, 9.17, and 9.18)

One of the most common reasons to order both transthoracic and transesophageal echocardiograms is to assess the heart valves and structures for infections. It's worth mentioning that patients who have low to intermediate suspicion for infection and have very good quality TTE may not need TEE for evaluation (just because we can, we should not always do as TEE is not a completely benign procedure). Right sided valvular vegetations are also often better evaluated with TTE than TEE.

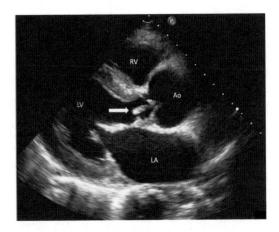

FIGURE 9.14 Parasternal long axis view showing aortic valve vegetation (*arrow*)

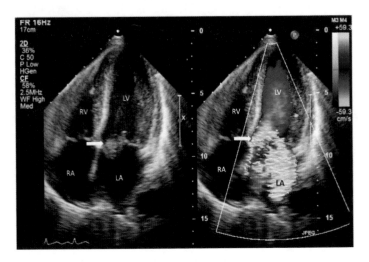

FIGURE 9.15 Vegetation (*arrow*) affecting the mitral valve with significant regurgitation (*right*) as a result of valve tissue destruction

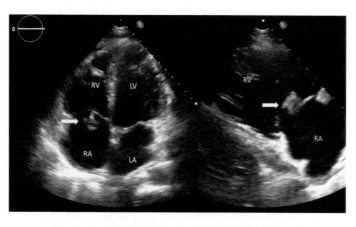

FIGURE 9.16 Apical four chamber (*left*) and RV inflow (*right*) views showing large vegetation on the tricuspid valve (*arrows*)

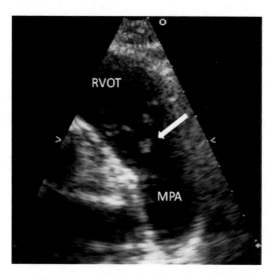

FIGURE 9.17 High parasternal view showing vegetation (*arrow*) attached to the pulmonic valve

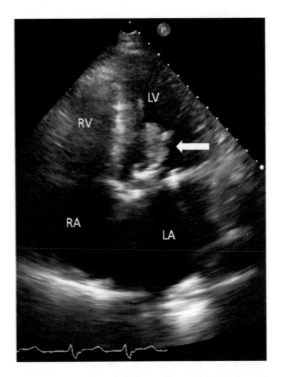

FIGURE 9.18 Apical four chamber view of fungal endocarditis (*arrow*) on a neochords of repaired mitral valve

References

1. Columbus MR. De Re Anatomica. Paris: Libri XV; 1559.
2. McAllister Jr HA, Fenoglio Jr JJ. Tumors of cardiovascular system. In atlas of tumor pathology, vol. 2. Washington, DC: Armed Forces institute of pathology; 1978.
3. Lam KY, Dickens P, Chan AC. Tumors of the heart: a 20 year experience with a review of 12485 consecutive autopsies. Arch Pathol Lab Med. 1993;117:1027–31.
4. Straus R, Merliss R. Primary tumor of the heart. Arch Pathol. 1945;39:74–8.
5. Elbardissi AW, Dearani JA, Daly RC, Mullany CJ, Orszulak TA, Puga FJ, Schaff HV. Survival after resection of primary cardiac

tumors: a 48-year experience. Circulation. 2008;118(14 Suppl): S7–15.

6. Silverman N. Primary cardiac tumors. Ann Surg. 1980;19: 127–38.

7. Bruce CJ. Cardiac tumors. In: Otto CM, editor. The practice of clinical echocardiography. Philadelphia: WB Saunders; 2007. p. 1108–3.

8. Bruce CJ. Cardiac tumours: diagnosis and management. Heart. 2011;97:151–60.

9. Gowda RM, Khan IA, Nair CK, Mehta NJ, Vasavada BC, Sacchi TJ. Cardiac papillary fibroelastoma: a comprehensive analysis of 725 cases. Am Heart J. 2003;146(3):404–10.

10. Maraj S, Pressman GS, Figueredo VM. Primary cardiac tumors. Int J Cardiol. 2009;133:152–6.

11. Fenoglio JJ, McAllister HA, Ferrans VJ. Cardiac rhabdomyoma: a clinicopathologic and electron microscopic study. Am J Cardiol. 1976;38:241–51.

12. Ganesh C, Shridhar A. A case of fetal cardiac rhabdomyoma. Int J Infertility Fetal Med. 2013;4:66–9.

13. Araoz PA, Mulvagh SL, Tazelaar HD, Julsrud PR, Breen JF. CT and MR imaging of benign primary cardiac neoplasms with echocardiographic correlation. Radiographics. 2000;20:1303–19.

14. Burke A, Virmani R. Tumors of the heart and great vessels in Atlas of tumor pathology. Washington, DC: Armed Forces Institute of Pathology; 1996. p. 1–98.

15. Lo Musio L. Nevoid basal cell carcinoma syndrome (Gorlin syndrome). Orphanet J Rare Dis. 2008;3:32–48.

16. Lambl VD. Papillare excrescenzen an der semilunar-klappe der aorta. Wien Med Wochenschr. 1856;6:244–7.

17. Hurle JM, Garcia-Martinez V, Sanchez-Quintana D. Morphologic characteristics and structure of surface excrescences (Lambl's excrescences) in the normal aortic valve. Am J Cardiol. 1986; 58(13):1223–7.

18. Deluca G, Correale M, Ieva R, Del Salvatore B, Gramenzi S, Di Biase M. The incidence and clinical course of caseous calcification of the mitral annulus: a prospective echocardio-graphic study. J Am Soc Echocardiogr. 2008;21(7):828–33.

19. Pomerance A. Pathological and clinical study of calcification of the mitral valve ring. J Clin Pathol. 1970;23:354–61.

20. Elgendy IY, Conti CR. Caseous calcification of the mitral annulus: a review. Clin Cardiol. 2013;36:E27–31.

Chapter 10
Estimation of Chamber Pressures

Dmitriy Kireyev and Judy Hung

Abbreviations

DBP   Diastolic Blood Pressure
EDP   End Diastolic Pressure
LA   Left Atrial
LV   Left Ventricular
P   Pressure
PA   Pulmonary Artery
RA   Right Atrial
RV   Right Ventricular
SBP   Systolic Blood Pressure
SP   Systolic Pressure

$$P_{\text{initial chamber}} = P_{\text{receiving chamber}} + P_{\text{lost/gained}}$$

D. Kireyev, MD (✉) • J. Hung, MD
Echocardiography, Division of Cardiology,
Massachusetts General Hospital, Boston, MA, USA
e-mail: dimonk5@yahoo.com; JHUNG@mgh.harvard.edu

D. Kireyev, J. Hung (eds.), *Cardiac Imaging in Clinical Practice*, In Clinical Practice,
DOI 10.1007/978-3-319-21458-0_10,
© Springer International Publishing Switzerland 2016

Left Sided Pressures

LVSP

In the absence of Aortic Stenosis: LVSP = SBP

In the presence of Aortic Stenosis: $LVSP = SBP + 0.7 \times 4U^2_{ASmax}$

LVEDP

In the absence of Aortic Regurgitation LVEDP = DBP

In the presence of Aortic Regurgitation:

$LVEDP = DBP - 4U^2_{AR\ end\ diastole}$

LAP

$LAP = LVSP - 4U^2_{MR}$

RAP

1. Use 10 mmHg [1]
2. Use IVC variation with sniff in Non-ventilated patients [2, 3]

    IVC diameter <2.1 cm; collapse with sniff >50 %: RAP 0–5 mmHg, use 3 mHg

    IVC diameter >2.1 cm, collapse with sniff <50 %: RAP 10–20 mmHg, use 15 mmHg

    Otherwise use 8 mmHg

RVSP

$RVSP = RAP + 4U^2_{TR}$

RVDP

In the absence of Tricuspid Stenosis: RVEDP = RAP

In the presence of Tricuspid Stenosis: $RVEDP = RAP - 4U^2_{TS}$

PASP

In the absence of pulmonic stenosis PASP = RVSP
In the presence of pulmonic stenosis PASP = RVSP − $4U^2_{PS}$

PAEDP

PAEDP = RVEDP + $4U^2_{PRED}$
Estimated   Peak   Systolic   Pulmonary   Artery
Pressure ≈ $10^{2.1-0.004(\text{pulmonary artery acceleration time})}$ [4]

Special cases:

Ventricular Septal Defect (with left to right shunt)
LVSP = RVSP + $4U^2_{VSDsystolic}$

Patent Ductus Arteriosus
PDA peak systolic gradient = Aortic peak systolic pressure − Pulmonary artery peak systolic pressure;
Peak gradients across PDA predict pulmonary artery pressures; high gradients predict low pulmonary artery pressures; low gradients predict elevated pulmonary artery pressure

References

1. Currie PJ, Seward JB, Chan KL, Fyfe DA, Hagler DJ, Mair DD, Reeder GS, Nishimura RA, Tajik AJ. Continuous wave Doppler determination of right ventricular pressure: a simultaneous Doppler-catheterization study in 127 patients. J Am Coll Cardiol. 1985;6(4):750–6.
2. Brennan JM, Blair JE, Goonewardena S, Ronan A, Shah D, Vasaiwala S, Kirkpatrick JN, Spencer KT. Reappraisal of the use of inferior vena cava for estimating right atrial pressure. J Am Soc Echocardiogr. 2007;20(7):857–61.
3. Rudski LG, Lai WW, Afilalo J, Hua L, Handschumacher MD, Chandrasekaran K, Solomon SD, Louie EK, Schiller NB. Guidelines for the echocardiographic assessment of the right heart in adults: a report from the American Society of Echocardiography endorsed by the European Association of

Echocardiography, a registered branch of the European Society of Cardiology, and the Canadian Society of Echocardiography. J Am Soc Echocardiogr. 2007;20(7):857–61.

4. Yared K, Noseworthy P, Weyman AE, McCabe E, Picard MH, Baggish AL. Pulmonary artery acceleration time provides an accurate estimate of systolic pulmonary arterial pressure during transthoracic echocardiography. J Am Soc Echocardiogr. 2011;24(6):687–92.

Chapter 11
Basic Congenital Heart Disease for Adults

Dmitriy Kireyev and Judy Hung

Atrial Septal Defect (ASD)

Types:

> Ostium Primum
> Ostium Secundum,
> Sinus venosus (both superior and inferior)
> Coronary sinus septal defect.

> Ostium primum septal defect (Figs. 11.1 and 11.2, Videos 11.1 and 11.2)

- defect in the group of atrio-ventricular septal defects appearing due to failure of septum primum fusion with endocardial cushion.

Electronic supplementary material The online version of this chapter (doi:10.1007/978-3-319-21458-0_11) contains supplementary material, which is available to authorized users.

D. Kireyev, MD (✉) • J. Hung, MD
Echocardiography, Division of Cardiology,
Massachusetts General Hospital, Boston, MA, USA
e-mail: dimonk5@yahoo.com; JHUNG@mgh.harvard.edu

D. Kireyev, J. Hung (eds.), *Cardiac Imaging in Clinical Practice*, In Clinical Practice,
DOI 10.1007/978-3-319-21458-0_11,
© Springer International Publishing Switzerland 2016

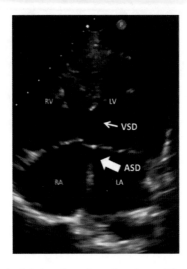

FIGURE 11.1 Apical 4 chamber view of patient with an atrioventricular canal defect showing ostium primum atrial septal defect (*thick arrow*) and corresponding inlet ventricular septal defect (*VSD-thin arrow*), Please note that the valve (which is a common valve) appears as if mitral and tricuspid valves are on the same level

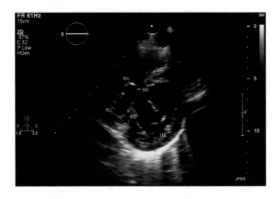

FIGURE 11.2 Apical short axis view showing a common valve in a patient with atrioventricular canal defect. *SBL* superior bridging leaflet, *IBL* inferior bridging leaflet, *LLL* left lateral leaflet, *RSL* right superior leaflet, *RLL* right lateral leaflet

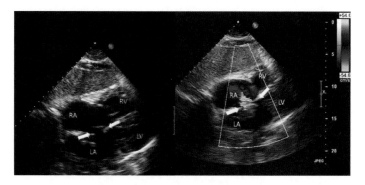

FIGURE 11.3 Subcostal views showing large ostium secundum atrial septal defect on the *left* (*arrows*) and shunt on the *right* (*arrows*)

- associated with AV valve malformation, cleft mitral valve and ventricular septal defects.
- due to complexity of the lesion it will not be discussed in this section.

Ostium secundum atrial septal defect (Fig. 11.3, Video 11.3)

- results from either poor growth of septum secundum or increased absorption of septum primum during early stages of development
- most common form of ASD
- commonly found in central portion of the septum surrounding foramen ovale.
- as left atrial pressures are higher than right atrial pressures, there is usually a left to right shunt early in the course of ASD which may stop and reverse the direction if pulmonary hypertension appears in cases of large shunts.
- TTE and TEE are useful in evaluation of size of the defect, it's location and feasibility of percutaneous device closure. Intraprocedural TEE is an essential part of percutaneous closure of secundum ASD (Fig. 11.4)

Sinus venosus septal defects (Fig. 11.5)

- Are divided in superior and interior

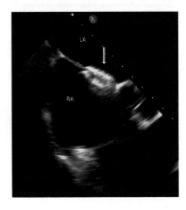

FIGURE 11.4 Transesophageal Echocardiographic view showing an Amplazer atrial septal defect closure device (*the arrow*)

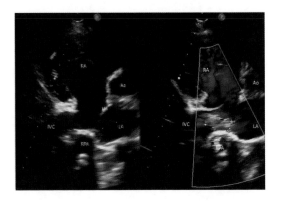

FIGURE 11.5 Right parasternal view showing Inferior Sinus Venosus Atrial Septal Defect with (*right image*) and without (*left image*) color Doppler. The jet of ASD is seen between 2 cross signs on the right image. *IVC* inferior vena cava, *IAS* interatrial septum, *RPA* right pulmonary artery, *Ao* aorta

- Occur due to abnormal insertion of superior or inferior vena cava (thus located in superior and posterior and inferior and posterior locations, respectively)
- Frequently associated with partial anomalous venous return

Coronary sinus septum defect

- Very rare
- Occurs due to incomplete formation of atrio-venous fold
- Often associated with persistent left superior vena cava

> Interesting fact: Scimitar syndrome: Combination of hypoplastic right lung, hypoplastic pulmonary artery, and anomalous arterial blood supply to the right lung and characteristically curved right pulmonary vein draining into inferior vena cava. The name appears due to radiographic resemblance of anomalous venous return to the shape of Middle-Eastern sword scimitar.

Echocardiographic assessment of ASDs:

- Type of defect
- Location
- Size
- Shunt ratio calculation
- Assessment of RA, RV
- Assessment of PHTN
- Imaging assistance in device closure of ASD.

Ventricular Septal Defects (VSD)

> Interesting fact: Ventricular septal defect was originally reported by Dr. Dalrymple in 1847. Glazbrook AJ. Eisenmenger's complex. *Br Heart J*. **1943;5:147–151**

VSDs are separated anatomically into muscular, membranous, supracristal, and inlet.

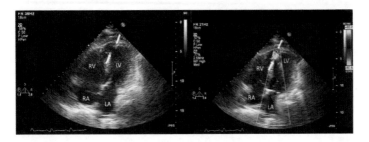

FIGURE 11.6 Off-axis apical four chamber views showing muscular VSD (*arrows*)

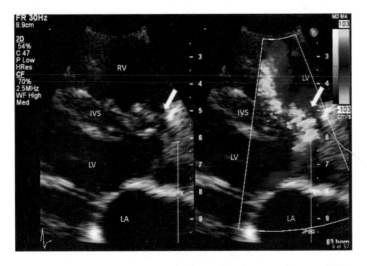

FIGURE 11.7 Parasternal long axis views showing membranous VSD (*arrows*). *IVS* interventricular septum

VSDs may be congenital or acquired (s/p myocardial infarction)

(a) Muscular VSD (Fig. 11.6, Videos 11.4 and 11.5)

- Most common VSD in neonates
- 90 % resolve within first year of life

(b) Membranous VSD (Figs. 11.7 and 11.8)

- Also known as perimembranous
- Most common type of VSD outside of infancy

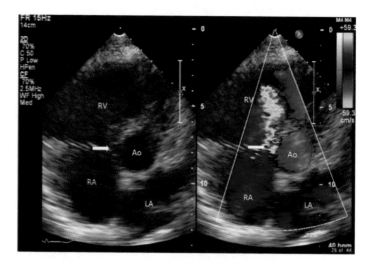

FIGURE 11.8 Parasternal short axis view showing membranous VSD (*arrows*). Please note dilated right ventricle

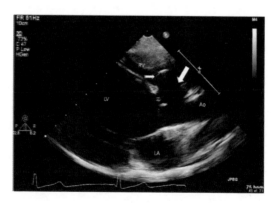

FIGURE 11.9 Parasternal long axis view showing patient with supra-crystal (cono-septal) VSD (*large arrow*) with aortic valve leaflet prolapse in the VSD (*small arrow*)

(c) Supracristal VSD (Figs. 11.9 and 11.10)

- sometimes called subpulmonic
- deficiency in the septum above and anterior to the crista supraventricularis beneath the aortic and pulmonary valves

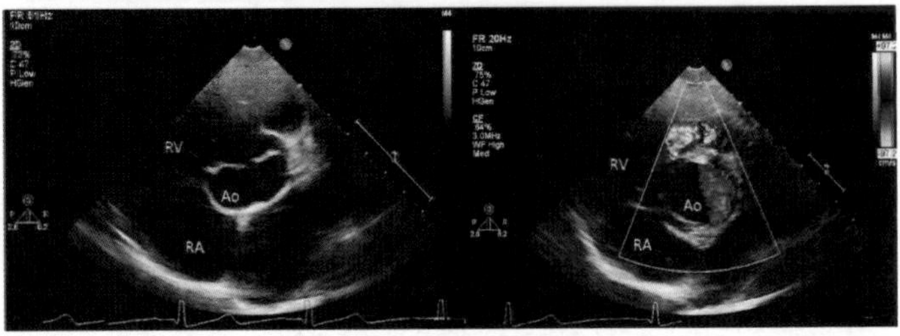

Figure 11.10 Parasternal short axis view showing patient with supra-crystal VSD and aortic leaflet prolapse. The right image shows the color Doppler image of the shunt

- lacks structural support of the right and/or the left aortic coronary cusp
- may cause cusp prolapse through the defect leading to aortic regurgitation (which is often progressive over time)

(d) Inlet VSD (Fig. 11.1)

- sometimes called atrioventricular canal type VSD
- associated with atrioventricular canal defects

(e) Malalignment VSD

- Anterior malalignment type associated with tetralogy of Fallot and truncus arteriosus
- Posterior malalignment type associated with interrupted aortic arch and coarctation

Echocardiography in VSD evaluation:

- assess the location and size of VSD
- assess the hemodynamic consequences (chamber enlargement, dilatation, RVSP estimation)
- Assess for other abnormalities which can be associated with VSD: ASD, patent ductus arteriosus, pulmonic stenosis, tetralogy of Fallot, transposition of great vessels, etc.

Patent Ductus Arteriosus (Fig. 11.11)

- Fetal connection between pulmonary artery and aortic arch
- Usually closes in less than 24 h after delivery
- Small PDA may not require intervention
- Large PDA associated with large left to right shunting and increased pulmonary pressure with progression to pulmonary vascular occlusive disease if not corrected

Echocardiography:

PDA is best visualized in parasternal short and suprasternal views

Evaluate: chamber size, RVSP, location of PDA, Qp/Qs

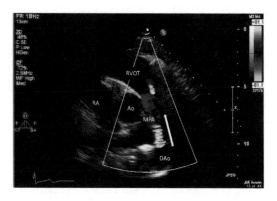

Figure 11.11 High parasternal short axis view showing jet from Patent Ductus Arteriosus (*arrow*). Note the smaller jet next to MPA label which is Pulmonic Regurgitation jet. DAo descending aorta, *MPA* main pulmonary artery

Ebstein Anomaly (Fig. 11.12, Video 11.6)

Ebstein anomaly was first described by German physician Wilhelm Ebstein in 1866. Interestingly, only 12 out of 272 articles that he published were about cardiovascular diseases.

Ebstein W. Ueber einen sehr seltenen Fall von Insufficienz der Valvula tricuspidalis, bedingt durch eine angeborene hochgradige Missbildung derselben. *Arch Anat Physiol* 1866;7:238–54.

vanSon JAM, Konstqantinov IE, Zimmermann V. Wilhelm Ebstein and Ebstein's malformation. *Eur J Cardiothorac Surg.* 2001;20:1082–5

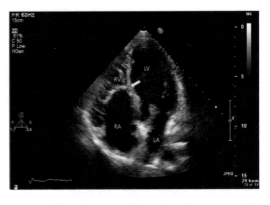

FIGURE 11.12 Apical four chamber view of patient with Ebstein anomaly. Note the apical displacement of the septal leaflet *arrow*. This change leads to atrialization of the portion of the right ventricle and anatomically smaller right ventricular chamber

- Ebstein anomaly consists of apical displacement of septal and posterior leaflets of tricuspid leaflets due to failure of delamination of septal and posterior leaflets, anterior leaflet is often elongated and redundant or tethered to right ventricular wall
- Clinical severity depends on multiple factors including the size of functional and atrialized portions of the RV, functionality of malformed tricuspid valve and associated clinical anomalies
- Associated anomalies include ASD, PFO, abnormalities of aortic or pulmonic valves, VSD. Left sided anomalies are present in up to 39 % of patients (Attenhofer JCT, Connolly HM, O'Leary PW, Warnes CA, Tajic AJ, Steward JB. Left heart lesions in patients with Ebstein anomaly. *Mayo Clin Proc*. 2005;80:361–8)

Cor Triatriatum (Figs. 11.13 and 11.14)

Interesting fact: Cor triatriatum was first described by WS Church in 1868. Church WS. Congenital malformations of the heart: Abnormal septum in the left auricle. *Trans Pathol Soc Lond*. 1868;19:188–99

- Cor triatriatum refers to presence of an extra membrane in the left atrium which separates the pulmonary vein drainage from the mitral valve and left atrial appendage
- Rarely this can occur in the right atrium and is referred to as cor triatriatum dexter.
- Functionally acts like mitral stenosis

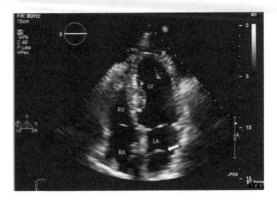

FIGURE 11.13 Apical four chamber view of a patient with cor triatriatum. Notice the additional membrane (*arrow*) dividing the left
atrium into 2 chambers

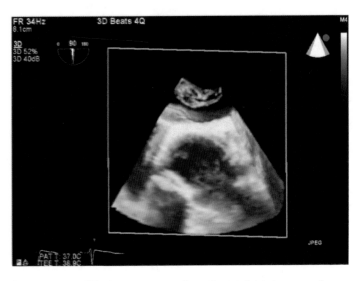

FIGURE 11.14 3D view reconstruction of cor triatriatum membrane
obtained during transesophageal echocardiogram. Note multiple
orifices allowing the blood to pass through one part of the divided
atrium into another

Tetralogy of Fallot (Figs. 11.15 and 11.16)

Tetralogy of Fallot, 4 components:

- VSD
- overriding aorta (anterior and rightward displacement of aortic root)
- pulmonary valve or infundibular stenosis
- right ventricular hypertrophy

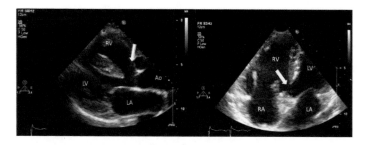

FIGURE 11.15 Parasternal long axis and apical five chamber views of the Tetralogy of Fallot. Please note the overriding aorta and the VSD (*arrows*)

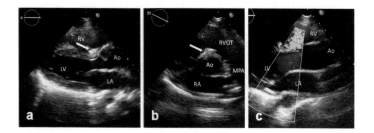

FIGURE 11.16 Images of a heart after repair of Tetralogy of Fallot. Parasternal long and short axis views (**a**, **b**) showing the VSD closure patch (*arrows*). Residual VSD can be seen by color Doppler in image (**c**)

Tetralogy of Fallot was first described by a Danish scholar Nicolas Steno in 1673. French physician Etiene Louis Arthur Fallot, after whom it was named, described it more than 200 years later in 1888.

Holomanova A, Ivanova A, Brucknerova I. Niels Stensen – Prestigious scholar of the 17th century. *Bratisl lek Listy*. 2002;103(2):90–3

Pentology of Fallot: tetralogy + either ASD or PDA

Associated lesions: stenosis of left pulmonary artery, bicuspid pulmonary valve, right sided aortic arch, ASD, PFO, abnormalities of coronary artery.

Echocardiography: diagnosis of the condition, assessment for repair, post operative follow up

Evaluate:

- Degree of aorta override (if >50 % of aorta overlies the left ventricle, diagnosis of tetralogy can be made while if >50 % of aorta overrides the right ventricle, the double outlet right ventricle is the correct diagnosis)
- The size of infundibular (+/−perimembranous) VSD
- Right outflow tract obstruction, quantity and location of stenosis as well as potential atresia
- RV size and contractility
- Determine the size of pulmonary arteries
- Look for anomalous coronary arteries (especially LAD crossing RVOT which may lead to potential intraoperative complication during corrective surgery).

Postoperatively (Fig. 11.17)

- evaluate VSD patch for residual VSD
- Evaluate right ventricular size and function
- Evaluate RVOT for obstruction
- Evaluate pulmonic valve for residual pulmonic stenosis and regurgitation

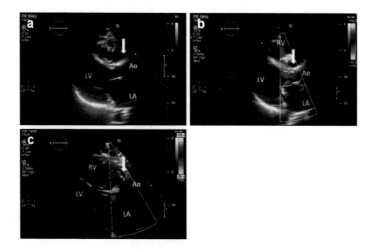

FIGURE 11.17 Parasternal long axis views of patient who has residual VSD along the VSD closure patch (*arrow*) after the repair of Tetralogy of Fallot. (**a**) parasternal long axis view, (**b, c**) parasternal long axis views with color Doppler showing residual shunts (*arrow* point to jets along the sides of the VSD patch)

Long term complications after initial repair of tetralogy of Fallot

- Ventricular tachycardia (look for RV dilatation, QRS >180 ms)
- RV failure secondary to pulmonary valve regurgitation (Pulmonary valve replacement is the most common surgery in patients with previously repaired tetralogy of Fallot)
- Severe TR
- Sudden Cardiac Death

Criteria for replacement of PV

- American College of Cardiology/American Heart Association guidelines from 2008 [1].

    - Symptomatic severe PR or severe PR with decreased exercise capacity
    - Severe PR and moderate to severe RV dysfunction and/or enlargement

- European Society of Cardiology guidelines from 2010 [2].
  - Symptomatic severe PR or PS
  - Asymptomatic patients with severe PR or PS and one of the following: decrease in exercise capacity, progressive RV dilatation, progressive RV systolic dysfunction, progressive at least moderate TR, RVOT obstruction with RVSP of more than 80 mmHg, sustained arrhythmias (both atrial and ventricular)

Transposition of Great Vessels

Interesting fact: transposition of great vessels was originally described by Matthew Baillie in 1797. Baillie M. Morbid anatomy of some of the most important parts of the human body. 2nd ed. London: J Johnson and G Nicol; 1797. p 38

- Aorta arises from the morphologic right ventricle while pulmonary artery arises from the morphologic left ventricle
- Can be either situs solitus (normal position of organs in the chest) or situs inversus (reversal of organ position in the chest)

D-Transposition of Great Vessels (Cyanotic Congenital Heart Disease) (Figs. 11.18 and 11.19)

- Atrioventricular concordance with ventriculoarterial discordance
- In simple terms: the patient has one loop of circulation where blood comes from right atrium to right ventricle to aorta and back to the right atria through the systemic circu-

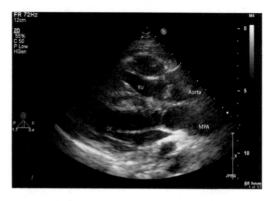

FIGURE 11.18 Parasternal long axis view of a patient with D-transposition of great vessels

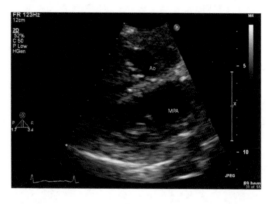

FIGURE 11.19 Short axis view of aorta and pulmonary artery in patient with D-transposition of the great vessels showing side by side alignment ("shotgun"). Aorta is on the top and Pulmonary artery is on the bottom of the image

lation, blood from left atrium comes to left ventricle to pulmonary artery to return to left atrium via the pulmonary circulation. In order to survive, such individuals need a shunt connection between those 2 circles of circulation (patent ductus arteriosus, VSD, ASD or patent foramen ovale).

Corrective surgeries:

- Mustard procedure (baffle SVC/IVC to mitral valve; Pulmonary Vein gets baffled to tricuspid valve), uses pericardium to create a single large buffle.
- Senning procedure creates a somewhat similar buffle within the atria using right atrial and interatrial septal flaps.

  N.B. both Mustard and Senning procedures are no longer performed (since 1980s)

- Arterial switch (also called Jatene procedure)
- Rastelli Procedure: used for transposition of great vessels with VSD: VSD is closed baffling LV to Aorta and RV to PA conduit is placed.

Echocardiography is used for continuous assessment of systemic and pulmonary ventricules, patency of the shunt and residual shunts.

L-Transposition of Great Vessels (Fig. 11.20)

- Congenitally corrected transposition of great vessels: transposition of the great arteries with ventricular inversion resulting in physiologically corrected flow: Systemic veins

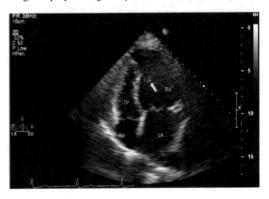

FIGURE 11.20 Apical four chamber view of L-transposition of the great vessels. Note the apically displaced atrioventricular valve on the right and faint outline of the moderator band (*arrow*)

to RA, RA across mitral valve into morphological LV from which arises the pulmonary artery; pulmonary veins to LA, across tricuspid valve into morphologic RV from which arises the aorta; note systemic ventricle is the RV
- Noncyanotic
- Associated anomalies such as VSD, Ebstein's anomaly, subpulmonary pulmonary stenosis and complete heart block

Persistent Left Superior Vena Cava (PLSVC) (Fig. 11.21)

- Most common variant of thoracic venous system
- Part of left superior cardinal vein which usually regresses and becomes ligament of Marshall. In cases where it fails to regress, persistent structure is called PLSVC
- Right Superior Vena Cava is usually present as well.
- In majority of patients PLSVC drains via coronary sinus into the right atrium; coronary sinus is dilated
- Patients are usually asymptomatic, findings are usually incidental

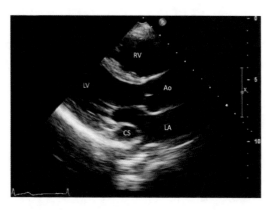

FIGURE 11.21 Parasternal long axis view of a patient with Persistent Left Superior Vena Cava. Please notice dilated Coronary Sinus (*CS*)

- Injection of agitated saline in the left antecubital vein results in microbubbles being seen initially in dilated coronary sinus and only subsequently in the right atria (in most common variant); Note: in case of injection into right antecubital vein the passage of microbubbles is normal
- Importance: PSVC complicates use of left subclavian vein for pacemaker/ICD wire placement and catheter placement. It is also a relative contraindication for the administration of retrograde cardioplegia during cardiac surgeries.

References

1. Warnes CA, Williams RG, Bashore TM, Child JS, Connolly HM, Dearani JA, Del Nido P, Fasules JW, Graham Jr TP, Hijazi ZM, Hunt SA, King ME, Landzberg MJ, Miner PD, Radford MJ, Walsh EP, Webb GD. ACC/AHA 2008 Guidelines for the Management of Adults with Congenital Heart Disease: Executive Summary: a report of the American College of Cardiology/American Heart Association Task Force on Practice Guidelines (writing committee to develop guidelines for the management of adults with congenital heart disease). Circulation. 2008;118(23):2395–451.
2. Baumgartner H, Bonhoeffer P, De Groot NM, de Haan F, Deanfield JE, Galie N, Gatzoulis MA, Gohlke-Baerwolf C, Kaemmerer H, Kilner P, Meijboom F, Mulder BJ, Oechslin E, Oliver JM, Serraf A, Szatmari A, Thaulow E, Vouhe PR, Walma E. Task Force on the Management of Grown-up Congenital Heart Disease of the European Society of Cardiology (ESC); Association for European Paediatric Cardiology (AEPC); ESC Committee for Practice Guidelines (CPG). ESC Guidelines for the management of grown-up congenital heart disease (new version 2010). Eur Heart J. 2010;31(23):2915–57.

Chapter 12
Ischemic Heart Disease

Dmitriy Kireyev and Judy Hung

Echocardiography is one of the most common imaging modalities used in evaluation of ischemic heart disease. It is used to diagnose coronary artery disease, assess consequences of coronary artery disease and give survival prognosis.

Electronic supplementary material The online version of this chapter (doi:10.1007/978-3-319-21458-0_12) contains supplementary material, which is available to authorized users.

D. Kireyev, MD (✉) • J. Hung, MD
Echocardiography, Division of Cardiology,
Massachusetts General Hospital, Boston, MA, USA
e-mail: dimonk5@yahoo.com; JHUNG@mgh.harvard.edu

D. Kireyev, J. Hung (eds.), *Cardiac Imaging in Clinical Practice*, In Clinical Practice,
DOI 10.1007/978-3-319-21458-0_12,
© Springer International Publishing Switzerland 2016

Diagnosis of Coronary Artery Disease

Stress Testing for the Diagnosis of Coronary Artery Disease

Exercise Echocardiographic Stress Test

- Patient exercises on treadmill or bicycle (Videos 12.1 and 12.2) with the goal of achieving at least 85 % predicted maximal heart rate (220-age of the person (bpm))
- Images are obtained at rest, at peak exercise (in case of treadmill version of the test the images are obtained right after patient steps off the treadmill) and during the recovery
- Parasternal long axis, parasternal short axis view, apical 4 chamber view and apical 2 chamber views are usually obtained
- ECG tracings are analyzed
- Assessment wall motion and contractility changes helps evaluate patients for presence of obstructive coronary artery disease. Degree of mitral regurgitation as well as changes in RVSP may be evaluated.
- Assessment for ischemic mitral regurgitation
- Stress test may also be ordered in order to evaluate valvular disease

Pharmacological Stress Modalities (Video 12.3)

- Used for patients who are unable to exercise or have low exercise capacity
- dobutamine echocardiography is commonly used
- dobutamine infusion (5–10–20–30–40–50 µg/kg/min at 3 min increments) is given to achive target heart rates
- If patient does not achieve target heart rate, additional administration of atropine (up to 2 mg) and ball squeezing maneuver can potentially augment the heart rate.
- Symptoms, ECG tracings and wall motion analysis is performed

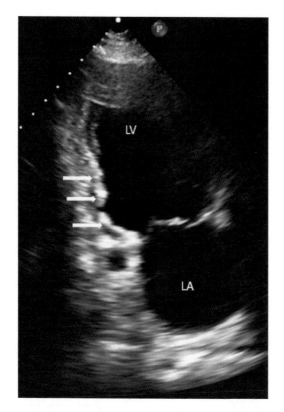

FIGURE 12.1 Apical two chamber view of a patient with inferior and inferobasal scarring (*arrows*) after myocardial infarction

Consequences of Coronary Artery Disease

Evaluate

- Wall motion abnormalities (Video 12.4)
- Scarring (Fig. 12.1)
- Aneurysm formation (Fig. 12.2)
- Mitral regurgitation (Video 12.5)
- Ejection fraction (even though Ejection Fraction does not have a linear correlation to the cardiac output, it serves as

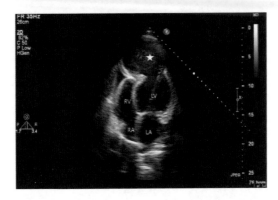

FIGURE 12.2 Apical four chamber view showing massive apical aneurysm (*star*)

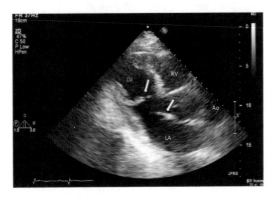

FIGURE 12.3 Modified parasternal long axis view showing ruptured posterior papillary muscle (*arrows*)

> a good approximation of the extent of myocardial dysfunction, potential prognosis and the need for both resynchronization and preventative defibrillation therapies)

- Consequences of previous or recent myocardial infarction:

  (a) Mitral regurgitation (including MR due to ruptured papillary muscles) ((Fig. 12.3), Video 12.6)

(b) Ventricular septal defects due to recent myocardial infarction (Video 12.7)

(c) Hyperdynamic left ventricular outflow obstruction (which is rare, but potentially life-threatening complication which is sometimes seen with inferior myocardial infarctions)

(d) Free wall rupture (Video 12.8)

Viability Studies

Dobutamine stress echocardiography may be used to assess myocardial viability through the evaluation of inotropic reserve of dysfunctional but viable myocardium. The increase in contractility induced by low-dose infusion may occur even in the absence of significant increase of blood flow. A 5–10–20 µg/kg/min doses with 3–5 min increments are usually used. Biphasic responce (initial improvement in contractility with lower dose with subsequent worsening at higher dose due to ischemia) increases positive predictive value of the test as well as recovery prognosis after revascularization.

Dobutamine stress echocardiography viability studies require higher percentage of viable myocardium for positive response when compared to Thallium-201 SPECT and FDG-PET modalities. (Baumgartner H, Porenta G, Lau YK, et al., Assessment of myocardial viability by dobutamine echocardiography, positron emission tomography and thallium-201 SPECT: correlation with histopathology in explanted hearts, *J Am Coll Cardiol*,1998;32(6):1701–8.)

Chapter 13
Cardiomyopathy

Parmanand Singh

Cardiomyopathy is a disorder of the myocardium associated with cardiac dysfunction. In this chapter, various forms of cardiomyopathy that are pathophysiological distinct are discussed.

Arrhythmogenic Right Ventricular Dysplasia (Fig. 13.1)

- Caused by progressive fibro-fatty replacement (dysplasia) of the RV myocardium.
- LV may be occasionally involved, with relative sparing of the septum.
- Patients may have ventricular arrhythmia of the left bundle branch morphology.

Electronic supplementary material The online version of this chapter (doi:10.1007/978-3-319-21458-0_13) contains supplementary material, which is available to authorized users.

P. Singh, MD
Division of Cardiology, Department of Radiology,
Weill Cornell Medical College, New York Presbyterian Hospital,
New York, NY, USA
e-mail: pas9062@med.cornell.edu

D. Kireyev, J. Hung (eds.), *Cardiac Imaging in Clinical Practice*, In Clinical Practice,
DOI 10.1007/978-3-319-21458-0_13,
© Springer International Publishing Switzerland 2016

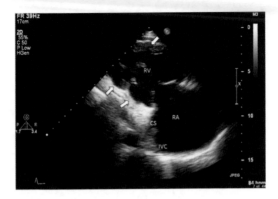

FIGURE 13.1 Right ventricular inflow view of a patient with Arrhythmogenic Right Ventricular Dysplasia. Note the right ventricular aneurysms (*arrows*). *CS* coronary sinus

- Familial linkage in approximately 30 % of patients (1st degree relative involvement).
- Characteristics EKG finding is epsilon wave.
- Morphologic features on imaging are hyperreflective moderator band, RV enlargement, RV dysfunction.
- RV aneurysms are highly associated with this disorder and their presence portends a worse prognosis.
- The presence of fat within the RV myocardium (as detected on MRI) is not a criterion required to satisfy the diagnosis.

Dilated Cardiomyopathy (Figs. 13.2 and 13.3)

- Characterized by dilation and reduced contractility of the LV or both the LV and RV.
- End-diastolic and end-systolic dimensions and volumes are increased.
- Systolic function indices such as ejection fraction, fractional shortening, systolic longitudinal motion of the mitral annulus, stroke volume, and cardiac output are diminished.
- Wall thickness can be normal.

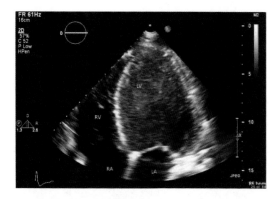

FIGURE 13.2 Apical four chamber view showing dilated cardiomyopathy. Note dilated and spherically shaped LV. Notice spontaneous echocardiographic contrast in the left ventricle consistent with low flow state

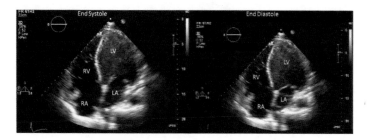

FIGURE 13.3 Apical four chamber view in systole and diastole showing poor ventricular function in patient with dilated cardiomyopathy

- LV mass can be uniformly increased.
- Secondary characteristics in this type of cardiomyopathy includes a dilated mitral annulus resulting in incomplete coaptation of the mitral valve leaflets and "functional" mitral regurgitation.
- Other secondary features include low cardiac output, dilated atria, right ventricular dilation and associated left ventricular thrombus.
- Interventricular conduction delay is common and results in intraventricular mechanical dyssynchrony.

- First degree family members should undergo screening with echocardiogram or cardiac MRI due to the high incidence (20–50 %) of familial dilated cardiomyopathy [1].
- PEARLS:
  - Pulmonary artery pressure estimated from the tricuspid regurgitation velocity is prognostics (velocity >3 m/s have a higher mortality).
  - Restrictive filling pattern (higher E/E' ratio, low DT) is associated with high mortality and transplantation rate [2].
  - Mnemonic ABCCCDE for some causes of dilated cardiomyopathy: Alcohol, Beriberi (thiamine deficiency), Coxsackie, Chaga's disease, Cocaine, Doxorubicin, Endocrine (hypothyroidism, thyrotoxicosis).

Hypertrophic Cardiomyopathy (Figs. 13.4, 13.5, and 13.6)

- Characterized by thickening of the LV resulting from a missense mutation in a gene that encodes the proteins of the cardiac sarcomere.
- Thickening or hypertrophy is usually asymmetric and can involves any segment of the LV, but often the ventricular septum.
- LV cavity size is usually normal or decreased.
- A subgroup of patients with a thickened interventricular septum may develop dynamic LV outflow tract (LVOT) obstruction.
- The increased blood flow across the narrowed LVOT produces a Venturi effect, whereby the mitral leaflets are drawn toward the septum, known as systolic anterior motion (SAM).
- Premature aortic mid-systolic closure can occur when aortic flow is interrupted by LVOT obstruction.
- Two-dimensional (2D) echocardiography provide excellent morphologic characterization.

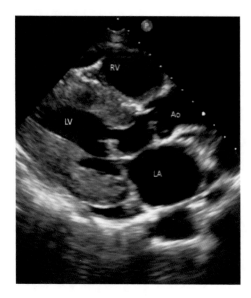

FIGURE 13.4 Parasternal long axis view of patient with hypertrophic cardiomyopathy (thickened septum and posterior walls). Please note the significant duration of SAM with LVOT obstruction with the M-mode in Fig. 13.5 (please note the anteriorly-directed motion of the anterior mitral leaflet towards the septum prior to LVOT obstruction [*white arrow*])

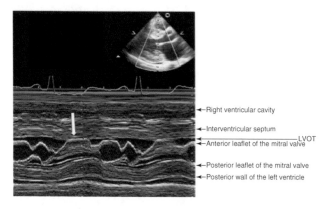

FIGURE 13.5 M-mode image showing dynamic LVOT obstruction (*white arrow*) in systole. Please notice duration of obstruction compared to the full cardiac cycle

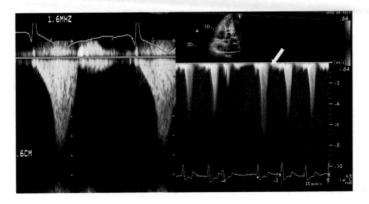

FIGURE 13.6 Velocity profile of dynamic LVOT obstruction in hypertrophic obstructive cardiomyopathy. Please notice the classical dagger shape of profile on the left and typical increase in the level of obstruction (*arrow*) after premature ventricular contraction (Brockenbrough-Braunwald-Morrow sign)

- M-mode echocardiography can assist in identifying SAM, premature AV closure and asymmetric septal hypertrophy.
- Contrast echocardiogram can be performed in cases of suspected apical variant hypertrophic cardiomyopathy.
- PEARL:
  - Ventricular thickness 30 mm or more increases risk of sudden cardiac death (~40 %) [3].

Left Ventricular Non-compaction (Figs. 13.7 and 13.8)

- Characterized by extensive trabeculation of the ventricular and deep intratrabecular recesses.
- LV cavity is typically enlarged and LV ejection fraction is decreased.
- In 2001, Jenni et al. (REF) demonstrated that patients are at risk for heart failure, sudden death, thromboembolic events and ventricular arrhythmia.

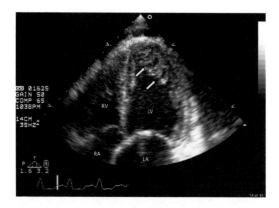

Figure 13.7 Modified apical four chamber view in patient with LV non-compaction cardiomyopathy. Please note extensive trabeculations of the left ventricle (*arrows*)

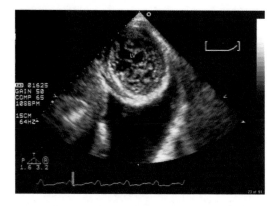

Figure 13.8 Short axis view of the apex of the patient with LV non-compaction

- On echocardiogram, end-systolic ratio of noncompacted to compacted layers great than 2.0 is diagnostic (delineation of these two layers is better visualized with contrast).
- With MRI, end-diastolic measurements of noncompacted to compacted layers are made, whereby a ratio of 2.1 is diagnostic.

- *Visualized affected segments*: With suboptimal echocardio-grams, contrast can be used to improve visualization of the number of potentially affected segments with greater sensitivity [4].
- *Correlation with clinical severity*: Amount of delayed trabecular hyperenhancement correlates with LV ejection fraction and is an independent predictor of LVEF [5].

Restrictive Cardiomyopathy

- Characterized by restrictive diastolic filling and decreased diastolic volume of either or both ventricles from an idiopathic nonhypertrophied inherent myocardial disease process.
- Typical morphologic features includes: normal LV systolic function, thickness and size with dilated atria (due to noncompliant ventricles).
- Typical features on Doppler:
  - Short DT, increased E/A ration >2.0 and decreased IVRT (restrictive filling pattern)
- Restrictive cardiomyopathy can occur as a results of infiltrative disease states such as hemochromatosis, amyloidosis and sarcoidosis.
- PEARLS:
  - Restrictive cardiomyopathy is not the same as restrictive hemodynamics.
  - Restrictive filling hemodynamic pattern can occur regardless of the underlying pathology, whereas restrictive cardiomyopathy is an inherent myocardial disease process that also produces a restrictive filling pattern [6].

Stress Induced Cardiomyopathy (Fig. 13.9)

- Also referred to as Takotsubo cardiomyopathy, apical ballooning syndrome, broken heart syndrome.
- Characterized by transient systolic dysfunction of the apical and/or mid left ventricular segments with hyperkinesis

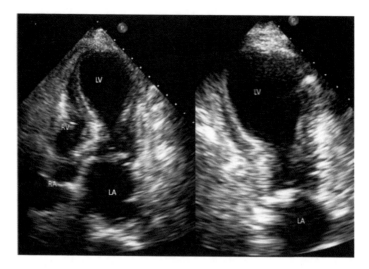

Figure 13.9 Apical four chamber (*left image*) and two chamber (*right image*) views of patient with stress-induced cardiomyopahy

of the basal segments, which produced a balloon-like morphology of the distal ventricle.

- First described in Japan but has since then been reported in non-Asian populations.
- "Takotsubo" is derived from the Japanese name for an octopus trap, which is similar in shape to the apical ballooning configuration of the LV in systole in the most typical form of this cardiomyopathy.
- Clinical presentation is similar to myocardial infarction, but there is no obstructive coronary artery disease.
- Frequently triggered by an acute medical illness, or intense emotional or physical stress.
- More common in women (~80 % of cases; mean age 61–76 years) than men.
- Pathogenesis is not well understood.
- Diagnosis is often made on echocardiography and/or MRI.
- Treat with standard medications for cardiomyopathy, including angiotensin converting enzyme inhibitors, beta blockers, and diuretics until there is recovery of systolic function, which occurs in within a month in the majority of cases.

References

1. Burkett EL, Hershberger RE. Clinical and genetic issues in familial dilated cardiomyopathy. J Am Coll Cardiol. 2005;45:969–81.
2. Rihal CS, Nishimura RA, Hatle LK, Bailey KR, Tajik AJ. Systolic and diastolic dysfunction in patients with clinical diagnosis of dilated cardiomyopathy. Relation to symptoms and prognosis. Circulation. 1994;90:2772–9.
3. Spirito P, Bellone P, Harris KM, Bernabo P, Bruzzi P, Maron BJ. Magnitude of left ventricular hypertrophy and risk of sudden death in hypertrophic cardiomyopathy. N Engl J Med. 2000;342: 1778–85.
4. Thuny F, Jacquier A, Jop B, et al. Assessment of left ventricular non-compaction in adults: side-by-side comparison of cardiac magnetic resonance imaging with echocardiography. Arch Cardiovasc Dis. 2010;103:150–9.
5. Dodd JD, Holmvang G, Hoffmann U, et al. Quantification of left ventricular noncompaction and trabecular delayed hyperenhancement with cardiac MRI: correlation with clinical severity. AJR Am J Roentgenol. 2007;189:974–80.
6. Ha JW, Ommen SR, Tajik AJ, et al. Differentiation of constrictive pericarditis from restrictive cardiomyopathy using mitral annular velocity by tissue Doppler echocardiography. Am J Cardiol. 2004;94:316–9.

Chapter 14
Echocardiography in Systemic Diseases

Dmitriy Kireyev and Judy Hung

Amyloidosis (Figs. 14.1 and 14.2, Videos 14.1 and 14.2)

1. Types of amyloid

   - AL – Primary amyloidosis, light chain deposition
   - AA – Secondary amyloid, deposition of part of acute phase protein (AA)
   - Familial amyloidosis – multiple types including transthyretin mutation (ATTR), apolipoprotein A-I and A-II, fibrinogen (AFib), lysozyme (L)
   - Beta-2 microglobulin. Beta-2 microglobulin does not get excreted by kidneys
   - Localized versions (many types) – including localized dystrophic amyloidosis of heart valves, senile atrial amyloidosis of the heart (Atrial natriuretic peptide)

Electronic supplementary material The online version of this chapter (doi:10.1007/978-3-319-21458-0_14) contains supplementary material, which is available to authorized users.

D. Kireyev, MD (✉) • J. Hung, MD
Echocardiography, Division of Cardiology,
Massachusetts General Hospital, Boston, MA, USA
e-mail: dimonk5@yahoo.com; JHUNG@mgh.harvard.edu

D. Kireyev, J. Hung (eds.), *Cardiac Imaging in Clinical Practice*, In Clinical Practice,
DOI 10.1007/978-3-319-21458-0_14,
© Springer International Publishing Switzerland 2016

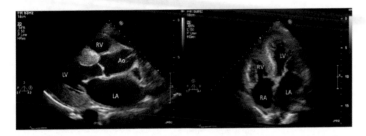

FIGURE 14.1 Parasternal long (*left*) and apical four chamber (*right*) views of a patient with Amyloidosis. Please notice thickened walls of both ventricles, speckled appearance of myocardium (better seen in the interventricular septum), biatrial enlargement and mild valve thickening

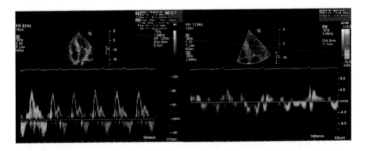

FIGURE 14.2 Mitral inflow pattern (*left*) and tissue Doppler (*right*) of patient with amyloidosis showing restrictive physiology

2. Cardiac involvement may occur in the following types of amyloidosis:

   - in AL and ATTR cardiac involvement is a major source of morbidity and mortality
   - AA

3. Presenting features:

   - Restrictive cardiomyopathy
   - Arrhythmias (both atrial and ventricular)
   - AV blocks and other conduction defects
   - Pleural and pericardial effusions
   - Ischemia from microvascular deposition of material

- Intra-cardiac thrombi (both atrial and ventricular)
- Low voltage on ECG and hypertrophied myocardium on echo

4. Echocardiography finding (note: they are very variable depending on stage of amyloidosis)

- Left ventricular thickening, concentric. RV is often involved
- Poor function of both ventricles
- Diastolic dysfunction
- Biatrial enlargement
- Speckled appearance of myocardium (note – this depends on gain settings)
- Valvular thickening
- Strain and strain rate abnormalities (long axis dysfunction is apparent even in early stages of amyloidosis)

Chagas Disease (Fig. 14.3)

Interesting fact:

Chagas' disease is named after Brazilian physician and bacteriologist Carlos Justiniano Ribeiro Chagas who discovered the disease. He names the pathogen Trypanosome Cruzi in honor of his friend and mentor, a famous brazilian physician Oswaldo Cruz, the founder of Oswaldo Cruz Institute where Dr. Chagas worked. Levinsohn R. Carlos Chagas and the discovery of Chaga's disease (American tripanosomiasis). *J R Soc Med* 1981;74(6):451–5

- Tropical parasitic disease caused by protozoa Trypanasoma cruzi
- Acute disease symptoms are non-specific and self-limited (fever, malaise, lymphadenopathy). However, small proportion of patients may present with myocarditis and pericardial effusions

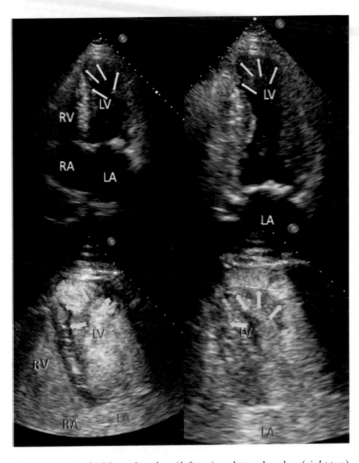

FIGURE 14.3 Apical four chamber (*left top*) and two chamber (*right top*) views and with LV contrast (*bottom*) of a patient with Chagas disease. Please notice apical aneurysm typical of this condition (*arrows*)

- Clinical symptoms develop in significant proportion of patients after one to three decades of asymptomatic infection
- Heart and gastrointestinal tract get affected

- Heart manifestations:

  Dilated cardiomyopathy
  High rate of LV apical aneurisms (with RV apex being affected in some patients)
  Segmental LV dysfunction
- Classification of Chagas cardiomyopathy – Brazilian consensus classification, all patients with abnormal ECG

  A. normal echocardiogram
  B1. abnormal echocardiogram, EF >45 %. No CHF
  B2. abnormal echocardiogram, EF <45 %. No CHF
  C. abnormal echocardiogram, compensated CHF
  D. abnormal echocardiogram, refractory CHF

- Main reasons for mortality: heart failure and sudden cardiac death

Loeffler's Endocarditis (Fig. 14.4)

- Eosinophilic myocarditis leading to myocardial fibrosis
- Restrictive cardiomyopathy
- Associated with hypereosinophilic syndrome

  eosinophilic leukemia
  carcinoma
  lymphoma
  drug reactions
  parasites

- Clinical presentation consists of 4 stages

  Necrotic
  Acute carditis
  Thrombotic stage
  Fibrotic stage

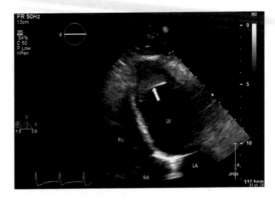

FIGURE 14.4 Off-axis apical four chamber view of patient with Loeffler's endocarditis. Notice the layered apical thrombus (*arrow*)

- Echocardiographic features (Fig. 14.4)

Localized thickening of the basal posterior wall of the left ventricular free wall
Apical layered thrombi

Libman Sacks Endocarditis

Nonbacterial endocarditis which is seen in Systemic Lupus Erythematosus and antiphospholipid syndrome

- Also called verrucous and marantic endocarditis
- Most commonly affects mitral or aortic valves
- Often occurs on the atrial side of mitral valve and aortic side of aortic valve
- May involve both atrial and ventricular sides of mitral valve
- More commonly causes regurgitation, but may cause stenosis

Carcinoid (Figs. 14.5 and 14.6)

- Carcinoid tumors are rare with majority located in the GI tract (most common in appendix and terminal ileum)
- Carcinoid syndrome: bronchoconstriction, facial flashing and intractable secretory type diarrhea

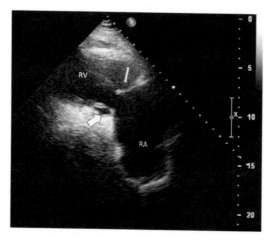

FIGURE 14.5 RV inflow view of a patient with carcinoid heart disease. Please notice thickening restrictive motion of the anterior (*thinner arrow*) and posterior (*thicker arrow*) leaflets of the tricuspid valve

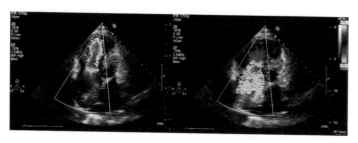

FIGURE 14.6 Color Doppler echocardiogram of patient with carcinoid heart disease. Please notice the presence of both tricuspid stenosis and tricuspid regurgitation

- Heart involvement is due to 5-hydroxytryptamine (5-HT), tachykinins, prostoglandins and other vasoactive substances released by tumor cells. Majority of substances are inactivated by lungs and liver.
- Echocardiographic features
  - Tricuspid and pulmonic valve and valvular apparatus thickening

- With the progression of the disease the valves get "frozen" in semi-open position with the combination of both stenosis and regurgitation
- Right atrium and ventricle show some degree of enlargement with right ventricular deterioration with the progression of the disease
- Left sided valve involvement may be present in patients with shunts allowing vasoactive substances to cross to the left side without inactivation in the lungs

Chapter 15
Echocardiographic Assessment of Aortic Disease

Asaad A. Khan

The aorta is the major arterial conduit which transports blood from the heart to the systemic circulation. It originates immediately beyond the aortic valve and is divided into an ascending aorta (initial ascending part) followed by the aortic arch (middle curve) and descending aorta (terminal descending part). The descending part continues through the hiatus of the diaphragm to become the abdominal aorta. The normal aorta is small, with a mean diameter of 3.2 cm (ascending aorta at the level of the right pulmonary artery).

Echocardiographic assessment of aorta aids in evaluation and management of acute (acute aortic syndrome) as well as chronic aortic conditions.

Acute aortic syndrome is the modern term that includes aortic dissection, intramural hematoma (IMH), and penetrating/symptomatic aortic ulcer. Advantages of transoesophageal echocardiography (TEE) for detection of acute aortic syndromes result from close proximity of the esophagus to

Electronic supplementary material The online version of this chapter (doi:10.1007/978-3-319-21458-0_15) contains supplementary material, which is available to authorized users.

A.A. Khan, MBBS, MRCP
Division of Cardiology, Massachusetts General Hospital, Harvard Medical School, Boston, MA, USA
e-mail: asaad.akbar@gmail.com

D. Kireyev, J. Hung (eds.), *Cardiac Imaging in Clinical Practice*, In Clinical Practice,
DOI 10.1007/978-3-319-21458-0_15,
© Springer International Publishing Switzerland 2016

the thoracic aorta and its ability to visualize both ascending and descending aorta and parts of the arch with high spatial resolution in real time. Although TEE requires esophageal intubation, images can be acquired at the bedside and immediately interpreted.

Aortic Dissection: (Videos 15.1, 15.2, and 15.3)

The aneurysmal aorta grows at about 0.2 cm/year. The larger the aneurysm, the faster it grows. Size continues to be a strong predictor of natural complications and a suitable criterion for intervention. Figure 15.1 shows a transoesphageal echocardiographic view of ascending aortic aneurysm.

Acute aortic dissection starts with a tear in the aortic intima following which blood enters the tear separating the intima from the media or adventitia, creating a false lumen. Propagation depends on BP and the pulse wave (rate of change in pressure/time) whereby high blood pressure and rapid ventricular contractions abet further migration. Complications such as malperfusion syndromes, tamponade, or aortic valve insufficiency are responsible for the subsequent clinical picture.

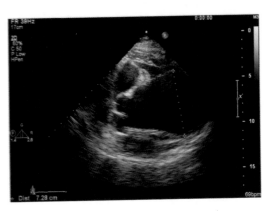

FIGURE 15.1 Transesophageal echo (mid-esophageal view) showing ascending aortic aneurysm (7.28 cm)

Two different anatomic systems, the DeBakey and Stanford systems, are used to classify aortic dissection [1, 2].

Aortic dissection is confirmed when 2 lumens are separated by an intimal flap visualized within the aorta. Tears can be identified and differentiation between true and false lumen is often easy and diagnostic with optional color Doppler flow mapping; intimal tear(s) can be localized in the majority of patients (Fig. 15.2).

Transoesophageal echocardiography is the echocardiographic imaging method of choice as it provides excellent visualization of ascending aorta, descending thoracic aorta and mechanism of aortic insufficiency. TEE is limited in assessing abdominal side branches and may be unpleasant for patients who cannot tolerate topical anesthesia and moderate conscious sedation.

Transthoracic echo (TTE) can be performed as an initial test for evaluation of aortic dissection if patient is very unstable and other modalities of imaging are not readily available. It can be performed at the bedside and can reveal acute aortic regurgitation and presence of an intimal flap (Fig. 15.3), although image resolution is not as good as TEE in general. It usually provides adequate visualization of aortic root and early part of ascending aorta. Suprasternal and subcostal win-

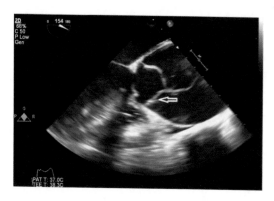

FIGURE 15.2 Transesophageal image showing an aortic dissection intimal flap (*arrow*) inside true wall

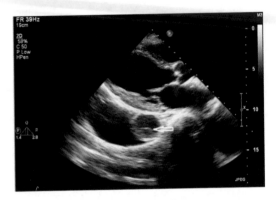

FIGURE 15.3 Transthorasic echo view of thrombosed false lumen of descending aortic dissection (*arrow*)

dows can provide limited but valuable data regarding aortic arch and descending aorta respectively.

Aortic Intramural Hematoma

Aortic intramural hematoma (IMH) is a variant of aortic dissection and is classified similarly. It is differentiated from aortic dissection by the absence of a detectable intimal tear and hence and hence, absence of continuous flow communication (Fig. 15.4).

The presence of a penetrating atherosclerotic ulcer on noninvasive imaging appears to have prognostic importance, being associated with a higher likelihood of progressive disease with medical therapy.

Exclusion of a dissecting flap or intimal disruption is a prerequisite for the radiologic diagnosis of aortic IMH [3]. Specific findings for aortic IMH on TEE include regional thickening of the aortic wall of more than 7 mm in a crescentic (primarily if nontraumatic) or circular shape (primarily if traumatic) and/or evidence of intramural accumulation of blood. The major finding on CT or MRI typically is a

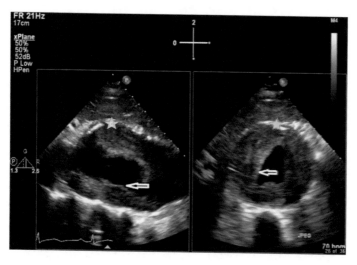

FIGURE 15.4 Biplane view of mural thrombus (*arrows*) inside abdominal aorta (*star*)

crescentic or circular high attenuation area along the aortic wall that does not enhance with contrast [4].

Penetrating/Symptomatic Aortic Ulcer

Penetrating ulceration of an atherosclerotic plaque often complicates an aortic intramural hematoma and can also lead to aortic dissection or perforation [5].

Echocardiography usually reveals an ulcer-like projection into the hematoma. Results of one study [6] suggested that penetrating atherosclerotic ulcers are almost always seen with a type B hematoma.

Overall, the European Cooperative Study Group and others have shown that TEE can reach a sensitivity of 99 % with a specificity of 89 %, positive predictive accuracy of 89 %, and negative predictive accuracy of 99 %, findings later confirmed in IRAD [7, 8].

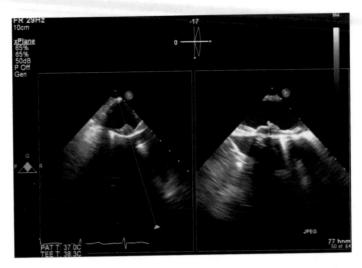

FIGURE 15.5 Measurement of atheroma thickness on a biplane view (Transesophageal image of descending aorta in a patient with recent cerebrovascular accident)

Role of Echocardiography in Chronic Aortic Conditions

In chronic aortic conditions, issues such as critical diameter expansion (Fig. 15.5), intraluminal thrombosis, protruding atherosclerotic plaques or vascular inflammation are in focus; serial comparison to previous imaging studies is often required. Transesophageal 3D echocardiographic imaging can provide a useful interface for monitoring these chronic aortic conditions. However, when repeat imaging is needed, MRI is most appropriate, offering 3D reconstruction and accurate dimensional quantification without radiation exposure.

References

1. DeBakey ME, Henly WS, Cooley DA, et al. Surgical management of dissecting aneurysms of the aorta. J Thorac Cardiovasc Surg. 1965;49:130.

2. Daily PO, Trueblood HW, Stinson EB, et al. Management of acute aortic dissections. Ann Thorac Surg. 1970;10:237.

3. Song JK, Kim HS, Song JM, et al. Outcomes of medically treated patients with aortic intramural hematoma. Am J Med. 2002; 113:181.

4. Vilacosta I, San Román JA, Ferreirós J, et al. Natural history and serial morphology of aortic intramural hematoma: a novel variant of aortic dissection. Am Heart J. 1997;134:495.

5. Tsai TT, Nienaber CA, Eagle KA. Acute aortic syndromes. Circulation. 2005;112(24):3802–13.

6. Ganaha F, Miller DC, Sugimoto K, et al. Prognosis of aortic intramural hematoma with and without penetrating atherosclerotic ulcer: a clinical and radiological analysis. Circulation. 2002;106(3):342–8.

7. Erbel R, Alfonso F, Boileau C, Dirsch O, Eber B, Haverich A, Rakowski H, Struyven J, Radegran K, Sechtem U, Taylor J, Zollikofer C, Klein WW, Mulder B, Providencia LA, Task Force on Aortic Dissection, European Society of Cardiology:. Diagnosis and management of aortic dissection. Eur Heart J. 2001;22: 1642–81.

8. Evangelista A, Mukherjee D, Mehta RH, O'Gara PT, Fattori R, Cooper JV, Smith DE, Oh JK, Hutchison S, Sechtem U, Isselbacher EM, Nienaber CA, Pape LA, Eagle KA, International Registry of Aortic Dissection (IRAD) Investigators. Acute intramural hematoma of the aorta: a mystery in evolution. Circulation. 2005;111: 1063–70.

Chapter 16
Basics of Agitated Saline Contrast ("Bubble") and LV Opacification Contrast Studies

Dmitriy Kireyev and Judy Hung

Basic Physics

When waves travel between two media, they may be transmitted, reflected and scattered. The reflection depends on the angle of incidence and difference in acoustic impedances between the media. Acoustic impedance (Z) is proportional to the density of the media and speed of sound in the particular media.

$Z = \rho c$ (where Z is impedance, ρ is density of the media and c is speed of sound in the media)

Air is an excellent contrast agent since it's density ratio to the blood is on the order of 10^5.

Electronic supplementary material The online version of this chapter (doi:10.1007/978-3-319-21458-0_16) contains supplementary material, which is available to authorized users.

D. Kireyev, MD (✉) • J. Hung, MD
Echocardiography, Division of Cardiology,
Massachusetts General Hospital, Boston, MA, USA
e-mail: dimonk5@yahoo.com; JHUNG@mgh.harvard.edu

D. Kireyev, J. Hung (eds.), *Cardiac Imaging in Clinical Practice*, In Clinical Practice,
DOI 10.1007/978-3-319-21458-0_16,
© Springer International Publishing Switzerland 2016

Types of contrast agents:

1. Agitated saline microbubbles
2. Encapsulated microbubbles. (Definity – lipid microsphere with octofluoropropane inside (1.1–3.3 μm), Optison – denatured albumin microspheres with octafluoropropane (2–5 μm), Levovist – lipid/galactose shell and air core – used in Europe)

Agitated Saline Contrast ("Bubble Studies") Use: Intracardiac Shunt Detection

1. Shunt detection (Fig. 16.1, Video 16.1)

    Agitated saline microbubbes can be used for right to left shunt detection. They create enough reflection to cause opacification of the right chambers of the heart and get dissolved while passing through pulmonary circulation (thus creating no contrast in the left heart).
    Method:
    Agitate 1 cc of air in 9 cc of air (using two 10 cc syringes and 3 way stop-cock) and inject rapidly into the venous circulation. In case of intra or extra cardiac shunts the bubbles will be noted in the left side of the heart. In case of

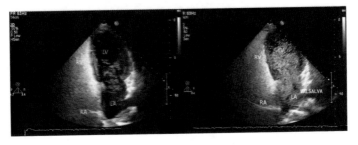

FIGURE 16.1 Agitated saline contrast ("Bubble") study in patient with PFO. The left image is done with rest, the right one is done during Valsalva maneuver. Notice the increased shunting with Valsalva maneuver

intracardiac shunt the bubbles usually appear in the left heart in 3–5 cardiac cycles after the opacification of the right heart. In case of intrapulmonary shunts the bubbles are more likely to appear more than 6 cardiac cycles after opacification of the right heart. In case of negative study repeat the study with Valsalva maneuver (bubbles are expected to be seen after the Valsalva release in patients who have the shunt which becomes more obvious with increased right sided pressures).

Note: in cases of significantly elevated left atrial pressure the detection of PFO/ASD by bubble study may be limited and color Doppler technique may be more diagnostic.

2. Diagnosis of persistent left superior vena cava (Fig. 16.2, Videos 16.2 and 16.3)

   Persistent left superior vena cava drains blood directly into coronary sinus. Thus, after the injection of contrast in the left arm vein it will first appear in coronary sinus and subsequently in right atrium. If the contrast is injected in the right arm vein, the passage of it will be normal with right atrial opacification prior to coronary sinus opacification.

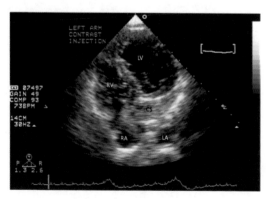

FIGURE 16.2 Apical four chamber view showing agitated saline injection via left antecubital vein. Note agitated saline entering right atrium and ventricle via dilated coronary sinus (*CS*)

Encapsulated Microbubble Contrast Study

Encapsulated microbubble contrast studies can be used for

- Left ventricular opacification
- Endocardial border evaluation enhancement (in studies with problematic visualization of more than two contiguous segments of the LV) (Fig. 16.3)
- Evaluation of the right ventricle and enhancement of tricuspid regurgitation studies
- Diagnose or rule out LV non-compaction cardiomyopathy or apical hypertrophic cardiomyopathy
- Diagnose or rule out myocardial wall rupture, aneurysm, pseudo-aneurysm (Fig. 16.4)
- Diagnose or rule-out intracavitary masses such as thrombus, tumor (Fig. 16.5, Video 16.4)

Contraindications to Contrast Studies

Definity   Know presence of the right to left or bidirectional shunt

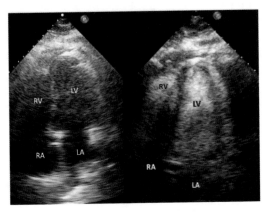

FIGURE 16.3 Apical four chamber views of patient with poor LV wall visualization (*left image*). Notice the significant improvement of assessment of LV walls with the contrast (*right image*)

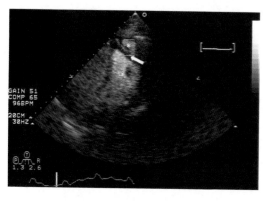

FIGURE 16.4 Apical two chamber view with use of contrast showing left ventricular free wall perforation (*arrow*) after left ventricular biopsy. Note the extravasation of contrast outside of ventricular cavity (*)

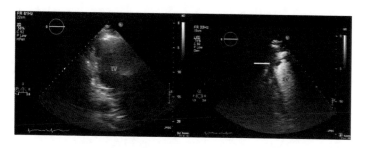

FIGURE 16.5 Apical 2 chamber view. The left image shows a non-contrast image. The right image shows the apical thrombus (*arrow*) which became apparent with the use of bubble contrast

	Hypersensitivity to perfluten (used in certain eye drops for glaucoma)
Optison	Known presence of right to left or bidirectional shunt
	Hypersensitivity to albumin, blood, blood products

Chapter 17
Nuclear Cardiology Imaging

Dmitriy Kireyev and Michael F. Wilson

Basics of SPECT

SPECT – Single Photon Emission Computed Tomography

Isotopes

Thallium 201 (Tl-201)

- Similar to Potassium (cation, monovalent) moves into cells via Na/K ATPases
- Decays by electron capture to Hg-201 (γ-rays 135, 167 KeV). 68–80 keV X-rays are emitted from Hg201: emission occurs due to rearrangement of orbital electrons to fill the vacant spot of captured electron.

D. Kireyev, MD (✉)
Echocardiography, Division of Cardiology,
Massachusetts General Hospital, Boston, MA, USA
e-mail: dimonk5@yahoo.com

M.F. Wilson, MD
Nuclear Cardiology and Cardiovascular CT Angiography,
State University of New York at Buffalo,
Kaleida Health Hospitals, Buffalo, NY, USA

D. Kireyev, J. Hung (eds.), *Cardiac Imaging in Clinical Practice*, In Clinical Practice,
DOI 10.1007/978-3-319-21458-0_17,
© Springer International Publishing Switzerland 2016

183

- Half life: 73.1 h
- First pass extraction: 85 %
- Rapid clearance from intravascular space with rapid monoexponential redistribution starting 10–15 min post injection
- Clearance: kidneys
- Produced in cyclotron

Technetium 99m (Tc-99m)

- m stands for metastable state
- Tc-99m sestamibi and Tc-99m tetrafosmin: Tc99m is attached to lipid soluble cationic substances. Tc-99m sestamibi: Tc-99m is bound to six methoxyisobutylisonitrite compound (MIBI). Tc-99m tetrafosmin is chelated by two 1,2-*bis*[di-(2-ethoxyethyl) phosphino]ethane ligands
- Tc 99m decays into Tc99 with the emission of several γ-rays including 140 KeV which is captured by the camera
- Half-life 6 h
- Lack of any significant redistribution
- Clearance: hepatobiliary system with GI extraction
- Produced in Molybdenum99/Technetium99m generator

Basic imaging acquisition (the most basic explanation which would not put you to sleep):

Photons (γ-rays) emitted from the patient's heart go through collimators (which allow photons from only certain directions to reach Sodium-Iodide crystal). The interaction with the crystal produces a flash of visible light which is detected by photomultipliers. Location of light helps determine the direction in which γ-rays travelled and amount of flashes is proportional to the amount of γ-rays entering the crystal. Computer reconstruction of signals allows 2–3D reconstruction of the heart.

Indications for Stress Tests

Stress tests are performed to diagnose and risk stratify patients who have known CAD or are at risk of having it.

Imaging supplementation is indicated in patients in whom regular stress test is non-diagnostic due to pre-test ECG findings making the test non-diagnostic, non-diagnostic regular stress tests results and patients who can not achieve target heart rate through exercise stress modalities.

Patients with left bundle branch block, permanent pacing, Wolf-Parkinson-White syndrome or severe LVH should be tested with the use of vasodilators in order to decrease risk of adverse events during the test as well as false positive results.

Diagnosis of CAD: stress tests should be used in symptomatic patients with risk factors of CAD or intermediate pretest probability of having CAD.

Risk Stratification

post myocardial infarction (prior to discharge, early or late)
prior to non-cardiac surgery
low to intermediate risk Acute Coronary Syndrome cases
patients with known CAD after either medical treatment optimization or revascularization

Contraindications

Absolute

- High risk acute coronary syndromes
- Symptomatic aortic stenosis
- Unstable atrial or ventricular arrhythmias
- Severe hypertension (SBP >200 mmHg and DBP >110 mmHg)

- Acute life threatening conditions: aortic dissection, decompensated heart failure, endocarditis, pericarditis, pulmonary embolism, intracranial bleed, etc.
- Recent myocardial infarction (within 4 days)
- Severe pulmonary HTN
- Rigor mortis (only in the absence of insurance)

Note: American Society of Nuclear Cardiology recommends NPO for 2h prior to the test – thus there is no need to keep patients NPO "after midnight". This may affect patients ability to perform well.

Stress Modalities

1. Exercise
   Patients should be preferentially exercised (via treadmill using Bruce, modified Bruce or either vertical or horizontal bike protocols) if there are no contraindications. Age should not be contraindication to exercise while the balance and ability to follow commands should. Do not forget that metabolic equivalents given by the machines for treadmill and bike modalities are not the same.
   Exercise test should be symptom limited (not by achieving 85 % predicted maximal heart rate $0.85 \cdot (220\text{-age})$).
2. Pharmacological vasodilator tests
3. Dobutamine test (should be used only in patients unable to exercise and having contraindications to vasodilator medications)

Pharmacologic Agents

Adenosine

- Acts on A2A receptor causing arteriolar vasodilatation in coronary bed
- Dose: 140 µg/kg/min for 4–6 min
- Half life <10 s

- Side effects: chest pain (non-specific), flushing, dyspnea, nausea, hypotension, bronchospasm, AV block
- Contraindications: Asthma with active wheezing, hypotension, advanced AV block, recent use of dipyridmole or dipyridamole containing products.
- Methyl Xanthines should be held for >12 h prior to the test

Dipyridamole

- Indirect coronary vasodilator
- Dose: 0.56 mg/kg infused over 4 minutes
- Side effects: similar to adenosine
- Contraindications: similar to adenosine (except it can be used in patients who are taking dipyridamole containing compounds)
- Use aminophylline to reverse effects of dipyridamole
- Random: be very careful while mixing the solution: yellow stains are hard to take off the white coat. Consider careful use of peroxide

Regadenoson

- A2A adenosine receptor agonist with lower affinity for other A receptors
- Maximal plasma concentration and pharmacologic response is achieved in 2–4 min
- Dose: 0.4 mg injected over 10 s with subsequent flush
- Side effects (generally mild and brief): shortness of breath, chest discomfort, dizziness, rarely AV block, etc.
- Use aminophylline to reverse the effect of regadenoson
- Contraindications: second or third degree AV block, bronchospasm, hypotension, use of caffeine containing foods within 12 h of the test (including decaffeinated coffee, tea, etc.), aminophylline within 24 h and dipyridamole/dipyridamole containing medications within 48 h of the tests

Dobutamine

- Stimulates β_1 and β_2 receptors. Increases heart rate and myocardial contractility. Blood pressure response is variable.
- For patients unable to reach target heart rate addition of atropine (given no contraindications) is beneficial.
- Dobutamine half life is 2 min
- Side effects include palpitations, arrhythmias, headache, chest discomforts, nonspecific STT wave changes

Contraindications

- Unstable angina or recent myocardial infarction
- Significant left ventricular outflow obstruction (HOCM, AS, etc.)
- Prior history of ventricular tachycardia or supraventricular arrhythmias with rapid ventricular response
- Patients with aortic dissections and aneurisms
- Severe HTN

Stress Protocols (Fig. 17.1)

- The goal of stress tests with nuclear imaging is evaluation of relative blood flow in different areas of the left ventricle at maximum hyperemia and comparing it to the relative blood flow pattern at rest.
- The stress test images consist of (Figs. 17.2, 17.3, 17.4, and 17.5):

  - Raw images (which allow basic visualization of the heart, the surrounding tissue and the motion of the heart due to patient movement which allows quality control check)
  - Short, vertical and horizontal long axis views (both stress and rest) which allow the comparison of perfusion and calculation of transient ischemic dilatation index

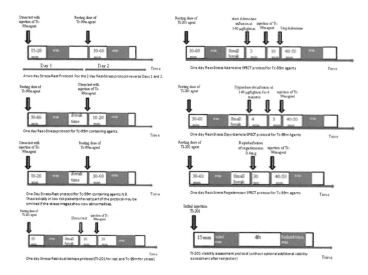

FIGURE 17.1 Most common protocols for stress tests and viability evaluation [1]

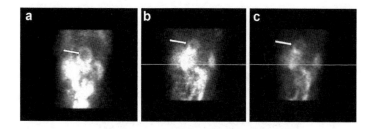

FIGURE 17.2 Raw images showing the heart (*arrows*) and breast attenuation in female patients (different angles of rotation are shown in **a–c**). Please pay attention to the dark shadows over the heart outlines

- Polar display: short axis views arranged from apex to lateral wall.
- Gated SPECT (to evaluate wall motion abnormalities and abnormalities contractility of the heart, and to calculate Left Ventricular Ejection Fraction through end systolic and end diastolic volumes)

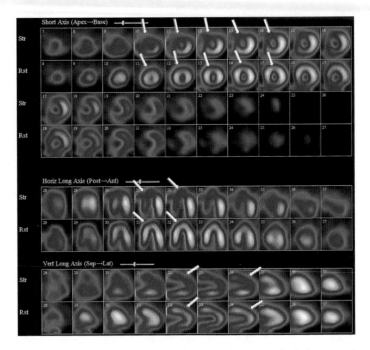

FIGURE 17.3 Tomographic images in short, vertical long and horizontal long axis views showing significant anterior ischemia (*arrows* point to ischemic regions in several view planes). Pay particular attention to the decrease uptake of anterior wall with stress (*Str, upper rows*) when compared to rest (*Rst, lower rows*)

There are several basic options for the protocols:

One day vs. two day protocols

Sequence of image acquisition: rest before stress or stress before rest

Single vs. dual isotope imaging

One day vs. two day protocols

Historically two day protocols have been preferred to avoid residual activity from first imaging to affect the second imaging acquisition. However, one day protocols have now become the more common. The two day protocol is preferred for obese patients (BMI >40) or women in whom significant

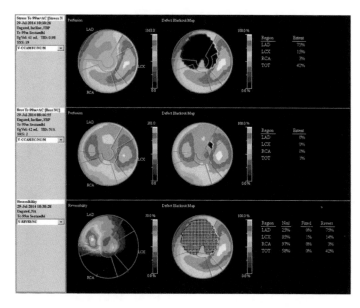

FIGURE 17.4 Polar display showing myocardial perfusion during stress (*upper row*), rest (*middle row*) and reversibility of ischemia (right lower image, meshed part of the image)

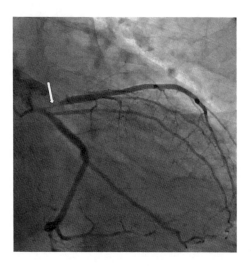

FIGURE 17.5 Coronary angiogram of the same patient showing proximal Left Anterior Descending Coronary Artery lesion (*arrow*)

breast attenuation is expected (thus potentially requiring a higher initial dose of radioisotope).

One day protocols are preferred due to practical considerations involving patient convenience, cost reduction and facilitation of decision making. This requires a combination of lower dose first imaging (rest or stress) and higher dose second imaging to differentiate between the first and second Myocardial Perfusion Images (MPI). Enough time for decay after the first dose is required prior to second acquisition and interpretation of MPI images.

Stress-rest vs. rest-stress sequence

- Low dose stress followed by high dose rest protocol

  Pros: possibility of avoiding extra images in cases where stress images are completely normal.
  Cons: increased radiotracer uptake by the myocardium during hyperemia requires either a longer delay between a stress and a rest acquisitions or a higher dose of radioisotope

- Low dose rest followed by high dose stress

  Pros: Less time is needed for acquisition of both scans leading to faster interpretation of tests
  Cons: necessity to perform both scans by default.

Dual isotope imaging

- Using Tl-201 for rest images and Tc-99m for stress images
- Is not commonly performed
- Was used more extensively during recent Tc-99m shortage
- Pros:
  Shorter duration of the test
  Ability to perform redistribution images (and thus assess viability) in patients with scars 4 h after injection of Tl-201
- Cons:
  Higher total dose of radiation to the patient.

Reporting Conclusion Details
(Use the Recommended Protocol Provided by Your Hospital If There Is a Preference)

Each report should ideally contain the following information

1. Indication for a test
2. One line summary of a patient including age, CAD (with details or risk factors) (Example): 57 y.o. man with CAD (s/p inferior myocardial infarction s/p bare metal stent implantation in 2005) presenting with new onset of chest pressure while jogging. Example 2: 40 y.o. woman with HTN, hyperlipidemia, DM and smoking presents with chest discomfort with exercise.
3. Doses of radioisotopes should be reported (Example: Myocardial perfusion images were acquired after intravenous administration of 8 mCi of Tc-99m Sestamibi at rest and 25 mCi of Tc99m Sestamibi at peak exercise heart rate).
4. Technical details of imaging should be reported and consist of the following: Quality Assurance Images (mention increased bowel &/or hepatic uptake anterior attenuation due to breast tissue, etc.)

   Technical description of images (examples: Tomographic images in short, horizontal long and vertical long axis view showed reversible inferior count reduction, example 2: tomographic images in short, horizontal and vertical long axis views showed mild fixed inferior count reduction consistent with male pattern and eliminated by attenuation correction). Mention transient ischemic dilatation index if increased. (?skip specific numbers since there is slight discrepancy between sources or not)

   Polar display interpretation +/– attenuation correction (example 1: Polar display shows inferior count reduction affecting 15 % of LV myocardium)

   Gated SPECT (mention LV cavity size if important, hypokinesis, LVEF). (Example: Gated SPECT showed dilated LV cavity, severe global hypokinesis and LVEF of 20 %)

Conclusion

- ECG interpretation with the information about the exercise (maximal fraction of predicted maximal heart rate and metabolic equivalents achieved needs to be reported). For patients who undergo pharmacological stress testing mention the medication which was used.
- Presence or absence of chest discomfort needs to be reported for exercise stress tests, for pharmacological stress tests it should be mentioned in cases of ECG changes.
- Interpretation of myocardial perfusion images and Gated SPECT (including normal reference of 50–75 % being normal in men and 52–77 % being normal in women)

Example of Conclusion

ECG positive for ischemia at 87 % PMHR and 6 METs of exercise

Positive chest discomfort

Myocardial perfusion images showed mild anteroapical ischemia involving 10 % of LV myocardium

Gated SPECT showed mild antero-apical hypokinesis and LVEF of 45 % (normal 52–77 % in women)

Viability Studies

Ischemic cardiomyopathy may occur in the presence of both reversible and irreversible myocardial changes including scarring, remodeling, hibernation and repetitive stunning. Revascularization may provide an improvement in heart function. The extent of viable myocardium may predict the potential improvement and need for invasive revascularization strategy in such patients.

Viable myocardium can be assessed by multiple different techniques including SPECT, Dobutamine stress echocardiography, Positron Emission Tomography and Magnetic Resonance Imaging.

There are multiple components of the viable cell system and the heart which may be assessed: cell membrane integrity, metabolism, mitochondrial activity, perfusion and contractile reserve.

Some of the common assessments and methods:

- Cell membrane integrity can be evaluated with Tl-201 SPECT
- Metabolism may be evaluated via scans using FDG (Fluorine-18 deoxyglucose)
- Mitochondrial activity may be evaluated using Tc-99m Sestamibi or tetrofosmin
- Contractile reserve may be evaluated via dobutamine echocardiogram or MRI
- Scar tissue extent may be evaluated by Gadolinium-enhanced MRI
- Perfusion may be evaluated by SPECT (as described in previous section)

Tl-201

Initial uptake of Tl-201 depends on perfusion. Redistribution of Tl-201 depends on functioning cell membrane (with functional Na/K ATPases)

Protocols

- Rest redistribution (rest images followed by up to 24 h redistribution imaging) (Fig. 17.1).
- Stress redistribution (stress imaging followed by 4 h redistribution images). This protocol is considered less reliable than the one mentioned above
- Late redistribution images obtained 18–24 h after the initial stress injection showed improved sensitivity of assessment for viable myocardium (no improvement over the rest-redistribution protocol was shown) [2]

- Reinjection protocol (second, smaller dose of radioisotope is injected to increase Tl-201 level with subsequent image acquisition). This protocol improves sensitivity of viability detection.
- Caveat: while Tl-201 redistribution showed viable myocardium, the absence of it does not completely rule out viability
- Nitrate enhancing: vasodilator increases flow in peri-infarct regions and increases delivery of radioisotope to the myocardium,

Tc-99m Sestamibi

- Passive diffusion across cell membrane
- Uptake and retention of compounds requires electro-chemical potential across mitochondrial and sarcolemmal membranes.
- Tc-99m sestamibi viability assessment is comparable to resting-redistribution protocol using Tl-201 [3].

References

1. Henzlova MJ, Cerqueira MD, Mahmarian JJ, Yao SS. Quality Assurance Committee of the American Society of Nuclear Cardiology. Stress protocols and tracers. J Nucl Cardiol. 2006;13(6):e80–90
2. Yang X-J, He Y-M, Zhang B, Wu Y-W, Hui J, et al. Assessment of myocardial viability in patients with myocardial infarction using twenty hour thallium-201 late redistribution imaging. Ann Nucl Med. 2006;20(1):23–8.
3. Udelson JE, Coleman PS, Metherall J, Pandian NG, Gomez AR, Griffith JL, Shea NL, Oates E, Konstam MA. Predicting recovery of severe regional ventricular dysfunction. Comparison of resting scintigraphy with 201Tl and 99mTc-sestamibi. Circulation. 1994;89(6):2552–61.

Chapter 18
Cardiac Computed Tomography

Jonathan Scheske and Brian Ghoshhajra

Technique

Interesting fact: CT was invented in 1972 by British engineer Godfrey Hounsfield of EMI Laboratories, England and by South Africa-born physicist Allan Cormack of Tufts University, Massachusetts. EMI was also a record label at the time that happened to have the contract of the Beatles and used the money from the massively successful Beatles albums to fund the development of CT. In a way we have the Beatles to thank for one of the greatest advances in modern medicine [1].

Basic Principles

Successful cardiac computed tomography (CT) depends on the ability to take reliable images of the coronary arteries, chambers, valves and other cardiac apparatus, despite the continuous motion of the beating heart. To accomplish this, scanning must be fast, synchronized to the cardiac cycle and have spatial resolution better than 1 mm [2]. Synchronization of the scan to the

J. Scheske, MD • B. Ghoshhajra, MD (✉)
Department of Radiology, Massachusetts General Hospital,
Boston, MA, USA
e-mail: bghoshhajra@mgh.harvard.edu

D. Kireyev, J. Hung (eds.), *Cardiac Imaging in Clinical Practice*, In Clinical Practice,
DOI 10.1007/978-3-319-21458-0_18,
© Springer International Publishing Switzerland 2016

cardiac cycle is termed ECG gating. Cardiac motion is minimal at end systole during isovolumetric relaxation and at end diastole as filling slows. Therefore, coronary imaging is performed during these phases. ECG gating and high temporal resolution also allow for functional imaging with cine acquisitions.

Patient Preparation

Hemodynamics

Generally only hemodynamically stable patients are appropriate for cardiac CT. In cases of instability, the benefits and risks of delaying or interfering with supportive and definitive treatment for diagnosis should be discussed directly with the radiologist [3].

Beta-blockade

Oral or IV administration; Target heart rate ≤65 beats per minute and regular. Adequate images can be obtained up to 100–110 bpm with certain high-speed scanners. Contraindications: SBP <90, asthma/COPD on beta-agonist, high degree heart block [2, 4].

Nitroglycerine

Coronary dilation improves diagnostic accuracy, particularly in the distal segments. Contraindications: SBP <100, critical aortic stenosis, Hypertrophic Obstructive Cardiomyopathy, narrow angle glaucoma, phosphodiesterase inhibitor use [5].

IV Access

High injection rate (up to 7.0 cc/s) improves image quality with high contrast density in the coronary arteries. ≥18 g IV in antecubital fossa ideal for most patients. In small patients <160 lb 20 g is likely sufficient as lower injection rate can be used. Central lines can be used if they are specifically rated for power injection [2].

Contrast

Required for evaluation of cardiac chambers, valves, coronaries, aorta and other vessels.

Contraindications:

Allergy

- 5 fold increased risk of reaction with history of allergy-like reaction to contrast [6].

Reaction Severity	Symptoms	Recommendation
Mild	Limited urticaria, itchy throat, nasal congestion, sneezing, conjunctivitis	Premedication not required
Moderate	Diffuse urticarial/erythema, facial edema or throat tightness without dyspnea	Premedication, consider alternate test
Severe	Diffuse or facial edema with dyspnea, laryngeal edema with dyspnea or hypoxia, erythema with hypotension, bronchospasm/wheezing, anaphylaxis	Premedication, consider alternate test

- Recurrent allergic-like reaction in 10 % of premedicated patients.
- No increased risk with history of specific allergy (i.e. Shell fish).
- Need for test should be confirmed, alternative test considered.
- Premedication recommended if history of moderate or severe contrast reaction requiring treatment
- Premedication strategies: 50 mg prednisone or 32 mg methylprednisolone by mouth, 13, 7 and 1 hours prior to contrast injection and diphenhydramine 50 mg by mouth, intramuscular or intravenous 1 hour prior to injection.
- In urgent situations, methylprednisolone sodium succinate 40 mg IV every 4 hours until contrast injection and diphen-hydramine 50 mg IV 1 hour before injection can be used. Optimal premedication effect is achieved 4–6 hours after steroid administration but effects develop as early as 1 hours after administration.

Moderate/severe renal dysfunction

– Risk of contrast-induced nephropathy rises with increased Creatinine (Cr) or decreasing glomerular filtration rate (GFR).
– Higher risk in diabetics, elderly, hypotension, dehydrated patients, patients on non-steroidal anti-inflammatory drugs and low body mass index
– No universally accepted guidelines by Cr or GFR
– Chronic stable renal dysfunction:

  • Cr 1.5–2.0 or GFR 40–60 consider prehydration
  • Cr >2.0 or GFR <40 strongly consider alternate test

– Acute kidney injury: no absolute guideline, strongly consider alternate test, prehydration and nephrology consultation
– Suggest renal function testing prior to CT with contrast:

  • Age >60
  • History of renal disease, including:

    – Dialysis
    – Kidney transplant
    – Single kidney
    – Renal cancer
    – Renal surgery

  • History of hypertension requiring medical therapy
  • History of diabetes mellitus
  • Metformin or metformin-containing drug combinations

Scan Protocol

Contrast Phases

Non-contrast

Calcium score calculation.
Often helpful to differentiate calcification, and high-density surgical material from contrast on subsequent phases.

Contrast Timing

Contrast injected into a peripheral vein returns to the right heart, circulates through the lungs, the left heart, and into the systemic arteries including aorta and coronaries. In healthy subjects this takes approximately 12–18 seconds; in patients with systolic dysfunction or valvular disease this can take up to 35 seconds or more.

Techniques for scanning with adequate contrast opacification include:

1. Set delay, usually 18–20 s
2. Bolus-tracking, opacification is monitored in the aorta and scanning is triggered as soon as a threshold is met
3. Test bolus, a separate, small contrast injection is given before scanning and opacification of the aorta is monitored to measure the time of peak opacification.

Test bolus is the most reliable but results in a small increase in scan time, contrast volume and radiation dose.

Gating

Gating is the process of synchronizing image acquisition or reconstruction with the cardiac cycle. Cardiac gating requires monitoring of the cardiac cycle using ECG leads. Scanners are programmed to sense the R-wave in the ECG tracing. Image acquisition can then be triggered at any desired point of the cardiac cycle, typically end systole or end diastole to minimize motion, or throughout the whole cycle to facilitate cine imaging.

Prospective Triggering

Images are only taken during specific, predetermined segments of the cardiac cycle. Patient selection: Slow, steady heart rate, ability to hold breath up to 15–20 s. Benefits: Less radiation. Challenges: Fewer phases of cardiac cycle available for interpretation. Longer scan time and breath-hold.

Retrospective Gating

Images are taken throughout the entire cardiac cycle. Patient selection: Higher heart rate with more variability, poor breath-holding/shortness-of-breath. Benefits: Shorter scan time/breath hold. More phases of cardiac cycle available for interpretation. Challenges: Higher radiation dose.

High-Pitch

Fast, spiral acquisition of the heart. Patient selection: Slow heart rate, poor breath-holding. Benefits: Low radiation dose, very fast acquisition. Reliable high quality images of all cardiac structures except for coronaries. Challenges: single phase of cardiac cycle available for interpretation, may be corrupted by motion artifact.

Angiographic

Images of the heart are acquired during peak arterial enhancement allowing detailed evaluation of the arterial structures.

Perfusion

Perfusion information is available on a typical angiographic phase. Contrast begins to reach the capillary bed 2–4 s after the coronary arteries. A myocardial perfusion deficit on angiographic phase scan is considered a resting perfusion defect; the culprit coronary lesion is considered hemodynamically significant to the degree that blood flow is limited even at rest [7]. Perfusion can be compared between stress and rest using two separate angiographic acquisitions, one with administration of adenosine or regadenoson.

Delayed

Additional images are acquired, without additional contrast administration, after the angiographic phase following a time delay. A delay of ~2 min is adequate for contrast to accumulate in areas with very slow blood flow, useful for:

Differentiation of late filling versus thrombosed false lumen in dissection

Differentiation of late filling versus intracavitary thrombus i.e. Left atrial appendage or left ventricular aneurysm

Extravasation of contrast from slow bleeding vessels

Identification of slow-filling subtle graft endoleaks

Enhancement of vessel wall in vasculitis

Further delay of ~7 min is adequate for contrast to accumulate in the myocardial interstitium, useful for:

Infarcted myocardium where the interstitial space is expanded by the presence of fibrotic scar tissue

Acute/subacute myocardial damage (infarct or myocarditis) where capillary permeability is abnormally increased.

Additional Considerations

Many features are specific to various manufacturers resulting in varying capabilities depending on the brand and model of scanner available. The following is a brief description of some of these features:

Slices

64-slice is the minimum recommendation for cardiac CT. Depending on the manufacturer, this corresponds to detector width ranging from 19.2 to 40 mm. The detector width equals the length of the patient scanned simultaneously. More slices/wider detector means a faster scan, less artifact, and shorter breath-holding for the patient [8]. At the time of this writing, scanners are available with 320 slices on a single source and 192 dual-source, covering 16 and 22 cm in a single CT rotation.

Dual source

Scanners with 2 x-ray sources allow extremely fast acquisition. The scanner collects twice the amount of information compared to single source, improving temporal resolution 2-fold. Coronary evaluation becomes feasible at higher heart rates.

Dual Energy

Reduces artifacts from metal such as coronary stents and can improve myocardial perfusion evaluation.

Indications for Cardiac CT

Indications for coronary artery calcium scoring, and cardiac CT angiography are listed below. For evaluation of coronary artery disease, pretest risk assessment is a major component of determining appropriate use of CT.

Pretest Risk Assessment

Low, intermediate or high risk is based on the Thrombolysis in Myocardial Infarction (TIMI) risk score for symptomatic patients and Absolute Risk Assessment Scores such as Adult Treatment Panel III (ATP III) or Framingham Risk Score in asymptomatic patients [3].

TIMI Risk Score

One point for each of the following:
– Age $\geq$65 years
– $\geq$3 risk factors for coronary artery disease (hypertension, diabetes mellitus, family history, lipids, smoking)
– Prior coronary stenosis $\geq$50 %

- ST – segment deviation on electrocardiogram at presentation
- ≥2 anginal events in the prior 24 hours
- Aspirin use in prior 7 days
- Elevated serum cardiac markers

For various TIMI risk scores, the risk of all-cause mortality, new or recurrent myocardial infarction, or severe recurrent ischemia requiring urgent revascularization at 14 days following presentation is as follows [9]:

TIMI risk score	14 day event rate (%)	Risk group
0/1	4.7	Low
2	8.3	
3	13.2	Intermediate
4	19.9	
5	26.2	High
6/7	40.9	

Absolute Risk

Low Risk

Defined by the age-specific risk level that is below average. In general, low risk will correlate with a 10-year absolute CHD risk <10 %.

Intermediate Risk

Defined by the age-specific risk level that is average or above average. In general, intermediate risk will correlate with a 10-year absolute CHD risk between 10 and 20 %. Among women and younger men, an expanded intermediate risk range of 6–20 % may be appropriate.

High Risk

Diabetes mellitus in a patient ≥40 years of age, peripheral arterial disease or other coronary risk equivalents, or the 10-year absolute CHD risk of >20 % [3].

Coronary Artery Calcium (CAC) Score: (Fig. 18.1)

- A screening test for patients without known history of coronary artery disease. Predictor of Major Adverse Cardiac Event (MACE) independent of Framingham Risk Score (FRS) [10]
- CAC score arranged into quartiles based on incremental risk of MACE for scores: 0, 1–99, 100–399, ≥400
- CAC most appropriate in symptomatic patients with Low Framingham Risk Score (10 year risk of MACE <10 %) and asymptomatic patients with Intermediate FRS (10.1–20 %)

Coronary artery calcium (CAC) score

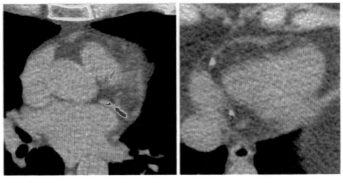

FIGURE 18.1 Non-contrast images from coronary artery calcium score study. Software identifies calcification with density greater than 130 Hounsfield units and applies color-coding by vessel. In the figure above, LAD is *red*, LCx is *blue*, RCA is *green* and non-coronary calcium is *yellow*. The subject above had CAC score 753, which is at the 99th percentile for subjects of the same age, gender, and race/ethnicity who are free of clinical cardiovascular disease and treated diabetes

- Positive CAC score is indication for medical management of coronary heart disease regardless of pretest probability of disease [4, 11]
- Sensitivity of coronary artery calcium for obstructive coronary disease 95–99 % [12, 13]
- Very high CAC score increases likelihood of non-diagnostic coronary angiogram [14].

Coronary CT Angiography (Figs. 18.2, 18.3, 18.4, 18.5, and 18.6)

- Detection of obstructive coronary artery disease: high sensitivity, 85–99 %, and negative predictive value, 83–99 %, in low and intermediate risk patients; specificity 63–90 %, positive predictive value 48–91 % [15–17]

Appropriate Use

- Stable angina: Intermediate pretest probability patients (10–20 % likelihood of CAD) [3]
- Acute chest pain: No evidence of ACS i.e. Negative troponin and no diagnostic ECG changes and low or intermediate pretest probability
- Prior testing: Uninterruptable or equivocal stress test.
- Pre-surgical risk assessment: Intermediate risk patients before intermediate or high risk procedures.
- Prior CABG or PCI: Symptomatic patients
- Suspected coronary anomaly
- Cardiomyopathy: Suspected ischemic etiology

Structure/Function Evaluation (Figs. 18.7, 18.8, 18.9, 18.10, and 18.11)

- Complex congenital heart disease, suspected mass/thrombus, or pericardial disease
- Alternative to technically limited MRI or echocardiography

Laft main (LM) and left circumflex
(LCx) coronary arteries

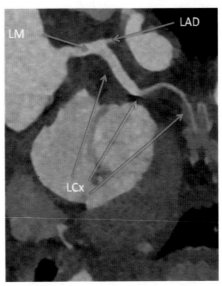

FIGURE 18.2 Curved multiplanar reformatted (cMPR) image of the
LM and LCx from contrast enhanced cardiac gated CT angiography.
The proximal LAD is seen branching from the left main coronary
and exiting the imaging plane. This non-dominant circumflex artery
quickly tapers as it travels down the atrioventricular groove

- Pulmonary vein evaluation prior to ablation.
- Coronary vein mapping prior to biventricular pacemaker
  insertion
- Evaluation prior to repeat sternotomy (proximity of vital
  structures to sternum)

Aortic Evaluation (Fig. 18.12)

- Suspected/Follow-up: Aortic dissection, acute aortic syndrome, vasculitis or aneurysm
- Planning for Transcatheter aortic or mitral valve
  replacement.

Right coronary artery (RCA)

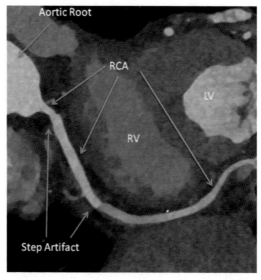

FIGURE 18.3 Curved multiplanar reformatted (cMPR) image of the RCA from contrast enhanced cardiac gated CT angiography. The vessel is smooth without athersclerosis. There are artifacts where the scanner moves from one slab to the next (step artifact or misregistration artifact), not confused for luminal stenosis

3D coronaries

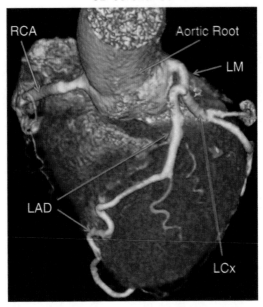

FIGURE 18.4 3D surface rendered image of the heart from contrast enhanced cardiac CT angiography. The left (*LM*) and right (*RCA*) coronary origins are seen arising from the sinuses of Valsalva and travelling along the epicardium

FIGURE 18.6 cMPR image of the LAD demonstrates atherosclerotic plaque with both calcific (*Ca*) and non-calcified (*NC*) component. The lumen narrows by approximately 90 % at the plaque, consistent with severe stenosis

Anomalous left coronary from right coronary artery

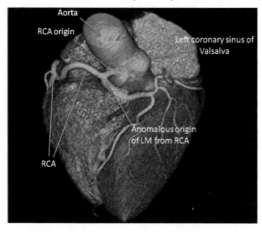

FIGURE 18.5 3D surfaced rendered image demonstrates abnormal origin of the left main coronary artery (*LM*) from the right coronary artery (*RCA*). It is readily apparent that no vessel originates from the left sinus of Valsalva, the normal location of the LM origin

Severe LAD stenosis

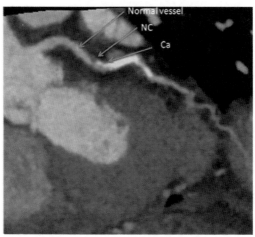

Axial	Coronal	Sagittal

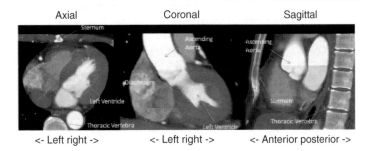

<- Left right ->   <- Left right ->   <- Anterior posterior ->

FIGURE 18.7 Axial, coronal and sagittal images of the heart. These are standard images reconstruction planes in CT throughout the entire body. Images are viewed as though looking at the patient form their feet (*axial*) face-to-face (*coronal*) or from their left side (*sagittal*)

Short axis and 2 chamber views

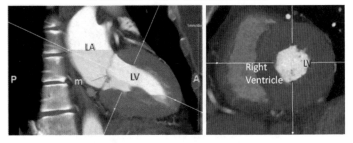

FIGURE 18.8 Left ventricular (*LV*) short axis view (*Left*) is parallel to the plane of the mitral annulus. LV wall thickness and motion are well seen. 2 Chamber view (*Right*) shows the left atrium (*LA*) and LV in long axis. The mitral valve (*m*) is also well assessed on this view

FIGURE 18.10 3 chamber/LVOT view demonstrates the relationship of the left atrium (*LA*), left ventricle (*LV*), Aorta (*Ao*), aortic (*AoV*) and mitral (*m*) valves. This view is useful for assessing LVOT obstruction, as can be seen in interventricular septal hypertrophy. (Interventricular septum – IVS)

4 chamber views

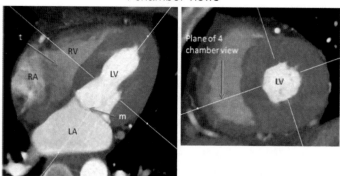

FIGURE 18.9 4 chamber view (*Right*) is perpendicular to the LV short axis view and shows the relationship of all four chambers: Left Ventricle (*LV*), Left Atrium (*LA*), Right Ventricle (*RV*) and Right Atrium (*RA*). Mitral valve (*m*) is seen, tricuspid valve is not well seen (*t*)

3 chamber/left ventricular outflow tract (LVOT) view

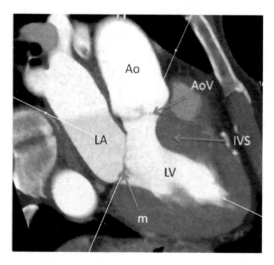

LV function short axis

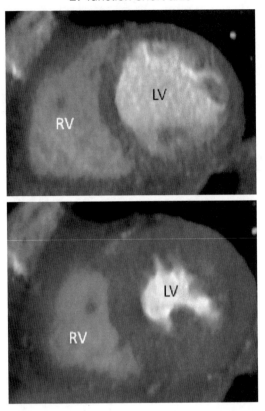

FIGURE 18.11 Selected images from contrast enhanced cardiac CT angiography in left ventricular short axis. Cine images were acquired throughout the cardiac cycle using either retrospective ECG gating or prospective ECG triggering with padding allowing functional assessment. Images demonstrate short axis views at end diastole (*upper*) and end systole (*lower*). There is normal thickening of the myocardium with >50 % thickening in all segments consistent with normal systolic function. Left ventricle (*LV*), Right ventricle (*RV*)

Aortic annular assessment prior to transcatheter aortic valve replacement (TAVR)

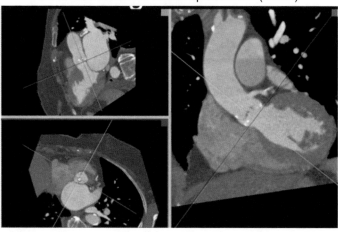

FIGURE 18.12 Multiplanar reformatted images from CT angiography performed in workup prior to TAVR. The plane of each image is represented by *colored lines*: *orange lines* for upper left image, *purple lines* for lower left image, *blue lines* form right image. The lower left image is the double oblique short axis plane of the aortic annulus, providing the most accurate measurement for sizing of the prosthetic valve. Important measurements for procedure planning include: annular diameter, area and perimeter; sinus of valsalva, sinotubular junction, ascending, arch and descending aorta diameter; and height of coronary artery ostia above aortic annulus. Important qualitative factors include degree and nodularity of aortic annular calcification and degree of aortic leaflet calcification. These factors help predictor procedural success

References

1. Alexander RE, Gunderman RB. EMI and the first CT scanner. J Am Coll Radiol. 2010;7(10):778–81.
2. Abbara S, Arbab-Zadeh A, Callister TQ, et al. SCCT guidelines for performance of coronary computed tomographic angiography: a report of the Society of Cardiovascular Computed Tomography Guidelines Committee. J Cardiovasc Comput Tomogr. 2009;3(3):190–204.

3. Taylor AJ, Cerqueira M, Hodgson JM, et al. ACCF/SCCT/ACR/ AHA/ASE/ASNC/NASCI/SCAI/SCMR 2010 appropriate use criteria for cardiac computed tomography: a report of the American College of Cardiology Foundation Appropriate Use Criteria Task Force, the Society of Cardiovascular Computed Tomography, the American College of Radiology, the American Heart Association, the American Society of Echocardiography, the American Society of Nuclear Cardiology, the North American Society for Cardiovascular Imaging, the Society for Cardiovascular Angiography and Interventions, and the Society for Cardiovascular Magnetic Resonance. J Am Coll Cardiol. 2010;56(22):1864–94.

4. Schoepf UJ, Zwerner PL, Savino G, Herzog C, Kerl JM, Costello P. Coronary CT angiography 1. Radiology. 2007;244(1):48–63.

5. Chun EJ, Lee W, Choi YH, et al. Effects of nitroglycerin on the diagnostic accuracy of electrocardiogram-gated coronary computed tomography angiography. J Comput Assist Tomogr. 2008;32(1):1–7.

6. Ellis JH. 2013. ACR Manual on Contrast Media, Version 10.1. 1-128. http://www.acr.org/~/media/ACR/Documents/PDF/ QualitySafety/Resources/Contrast%20Manual/2015_Contrast_ Media.pdf.

7. Blankstein R, Shturman LD, Rogers IS, et al. Adenosine-induced stress myocardial perfusion imaging using dual-source cardiac computed tomography. J Am Coll Cardiol. 2009;54(12):1072–84.

8. Goldman LW. Principles of CT: multislice CT. J Nucl Med Technol. 2008;36(2):57–68.

9. Antman EM, Cohen M, Bernink PJLM, et al. The TIMI risk score for unstable angina/non–ST elevation MI: a method for prognostication and therapeutic decision making. JAMA. 2000;284(7):835–42.

10. Greenland P, Bonow RO, Brundage BH, et al. ACCF/AHA 2007 clinical expert consensus document on coronary artery calcium scoring by computed tomography in global cardiovascular risk assessment and in evaluation of patients with chest pain: a report of the American College of Cardiology Foundation Clinical Expert Consensus Task Force (ACCF/AHA Writing Committee to Update the 2000 Expert Consensus Document on Electron Beam Computed Tomography) developed in collaboration with the Society of Atherosclerosis Imaging and Prevention and the Society of Cardiovascular Computed Tomography. J Am Coll Cardiol. 2007;49(3):378–402.

11. Parikh S, Budoff MJ. Calcium scoring and cardiac computed tomography in 2014. Cardiol Clin. 2014;32(3):419–27.
12. Budoff MJ, Diamond GA, Raggi P, et al. Continuous probabilistic prediction of angiographically significant coronary artery disease using electron beam tomography. Circulation. 2002; 105(15):1791–6.
13. Haberl R, Becker A, Leber A, et al. Correlation of coronary calcification and angiographically documented stenoses in patients with suspected coronary artery disease: results of 1,764 patients. J Am Coll Cardiol. 2001;37(2):451–7.
14. Pundziute G, Schuijf J, Jukema J, et al. Impact of coronary calcium score on diagnostic accuracy of multislice computed tomography coronary angiography for detection of coronary artery disease. J Nucl Cardiol. 2007;14(1):36–43.
15. Budoff MJ, Dowe D, Jollis JG, et al. Diagnostic performance of 64-multidetector row coronary computed tomographic angiography for evaluation of coronary artery stenosis in individuals without known coronary artery disease: results from the prospective multicenter ACCURACY (Assessment by Coronary Computed Tomographic Angiography of Individuals Undergoing Invasive Coronary Angiography) trial. J Am Coll Cardiol. 2008;52(21):1724–32.
16. Miller JM, Rochitte CE, Dewey M, et al. Diagnostic performance of coronary angiography by 64-row CT. N Engl J Med. 2008;359(22):2324–36.
17. Meijboom WB, Meijs MFL, Schuijf JD, et al. Diagnostic accuracy of 64-slice computed tomography coronary angiography: a prospective, multicenter, multivendor study. J Am Coll Cardiol. 2008;52(25):2135–44.

Chapter 19
Cardiac Magnetic Resonance (CMR) Imaging

Marcello Panagia, Jonathan Scheske, Brian Ghoshhajra, and Sanjeev A. Francis

Magnet Considerations and Safety

- Magnet is "always on" and therefore ANY ferromagnetic material entering the magnet room will be attracted to the bore of the magnet and potentially be a lethal projectile.
- Magnetic field strength is measured in Tesla (T) and typical commercial scanners for CMR are 1.0 T, 1.5 T and 3.0 T.

  - Higher field strengths provide better signal to noise (SNR) but potential for more artifacts.

- Ferromagnetic devices and implants should be screened prior to the CMR study.

M. Panagia, MD, PhD (✉)
Cardiology Division, Massachusetts General Hospital,
Boston, MA, USA
e-mail: a.mpanagia@nmr.mgh.harvard.edu

J. Scheske, MD • B. Ghoshhajra, MD
Department of Radiology, Massachusetts General Hospital,
Boston, MA, USA

S.A. Francis, MD
Cardio-Oncology Program, Cardiac MRI/CT Program,
Massachusetts General Hospital, Boston, MA, USA

D. Kireyev, J. Hung (eds.), *Cardiac Imaging in Clinical Practice*, In Clinical Practice,
DOI 10.1007/978-3-319-21458-0_19,
© Springer International Publishing Switzerland 2016

- Devices are generally divided into MR unsafe (e.g. insulin pumps, most ICD's, metal foreign bodies in eyes), MR conditional (most heart valves, coronary stents, prosthetic joints) and MR safe.
- Each device undergoes separate testing and you can check MR compatibility at www.mrisafety.com
- Weakly ferromagnetic devices (heart valves, some stents) generally undergo greater mechanical forces due to heart motion than to magnetic forces. If there is no urgency to the MR study waiting approximately 6 weeks after implantation can be considered. For some devices (i.e. coronary stents) there is sufficient safety data to allow patients to be scanned without delay.
- Permanent pacemakers and ICD's are currently labeled as MR unsafe and can undergo damage, movement, inhibition of pacing output, activation of tachyarrhythmia therapies and heating of electrode leads. CMR compatible pacemakers are being developed.
- Temporary pacemakers or hemodynamic catheters that contain conducting wires are generally considered MR unsafe.
- Gadolinium (Gd) contrast agents have been associated with allergic reactions (hives, SOB) as well as anaphylaxis though this occurs at a lower rate compared to iodinated contrast.
- Use of Gd in end stage renal disease (ESRD) has been associated with a risk for nephrogenic systemic fibrosis (NSF) (3–5 %) that can be fatal.
- Use of Gd contrast in patients with eGFR <30 mL/min must be approached with caution.

  – Should consider post-procedure hemodialysis in patients with ESRD if they receive Gd contrast (Table 19.1).

Basic MRI Physics

- Can "tune" CMR magnet coils to different frequencies in order to image different paramagnetic nuclei (^{31}P, ^{23}Na, ^{13}C, ^{1}H).

TABLE 19.1 Advantages and disadvantages of CMR

Advantages	Disadvantages
Non invasive	Contraindicated in patients with certain brain aneurysm clips, ferromagnetic shrapnel in eyes, pacemakers and ICDs
No ionizing radiation (useful for serial follow up studies especially in pediatric populations)	ECG and respiratory gating can be challenging creating motion artifacts
No radioactive isotope or iodinated contrast	Acquisition times can be long depending on purpose of study
Images can be acquired in any tomographic plane in 3D without restrictions from body habitus	Patient tolerance (length of scan, claustrophobia, ability to breath hold)
High spatial and temporal resolution	Gd based contrast associated with NSF in patients with low GFR
Many imaging techniques to assess and quantify multiple aspects of cardiac anatomy and function in one scan session	Significant expertise is necessary for a high quality scan (operator dependent) and refined interpretation of results
Fast-paced hardware, software and sequence development improving scanning technology	
Increasing number of indications for use	

- Proton imaging is most commonly used clinically because of high natural abundance in water and lipid molecules (creates high SNR).

• In the presence of the static magnetic field (B_0), a proportion of the protons will align themselves in the direction of the magnetic field forming a net magnetization.

- Size of net magnetization determines the signal intensity that can be used for image formation.

  • Higher signal intensity means better image quality (hence better image quality at higher field strengths) but also increased susceptibility to certain artifacts.

• Protons will "precess" around the axis of B_0 and the frequency of precession is dependent on the inherent property of the nuclei being imaged and the field strength.
• The angle of alignment with B_0 and phase coherence (whether protons are spinning at the same frequency) can be perturbed with radiofrequency (rf) pulse sequences.
• Applying controlled rf pulse sequences at different spatial locations allows you to take advantage of the inherent magnetic properties of different tissues (and pathologic states) producing tissue contrast.

  - After a pulse sequence is applied, the protons in the tissue are "excited" (out of alignment with B_0).

    • As the protons return to baseline alignment (relaxation), the energy released can be recorded by receiving coils and the signal produced can be temporally and spatially encoded to produce an image.

  - By varying characteristics of the rf pulse sequence (e.g. repetition time, echo time, flip angle etc.) you can create unique pulse sequences and probe tissue characteristics.

    • This is a unique feature of MRI.

• After an rf pulse is applied, the system begins to relax and there are two kinds of relaxation.

  - T1 relaxation (longitudinal relaxation) is responsible for the realignment of the proton spins with B_0 (after the rf pulse has created an angle between the magnetic moment of the proton and B_0).

    • The flip angle is the angle that is generate by the rf pulse between the magnetic moment of the proton and B_0.

- T1 relaxation is an exponential process that is tissue specific.
- The faster the relaxation the shorter the T1 constant (time it takes for the longitudinal magnetization to return to 63 % of its equilibrium value).

  - Fat has a short T1 and water has a longer T1.
  - Inflammatory processes will increase T1.
  - Gd contrast shortens T1.

- By taking advantage of intrinsic T1 properties of tissues, you can create pulse sequences that are T1 weighted to bring out tissue contrast and tissue pathology.

- T2 relaxation (transverse relaxation or spin-spin relaxation) is the loss of phase coherence of protons after the rf pulse has initially caused them to rotate together.

  - Immediately after the rf pulse, the spins are said to be "in phase."
  - Over time rotating spins will interact with each other and with B_0 causing de-phasing.
  - T2 relaxation is also tissue specific and pathology specific.
  - T2 is also an exponential process with a time constant that represents the time it takes for the magnetization signal to decay (de-phase) to 37 % of the value immediately after the rf pulse.

    - Muscle has a short T2 value, but as water content is increased (e.g. edema) the T2 value also increases.

  - T2* is the time constant (relaxation) that results from spin-spin interactions (T2) as well as magnetic field inhomogeneity.

    - Although T2 decay is irreversible, the additional decay caused by magnetic field inhomogeneity can be reversed with a 180° refocusing pulse.

Image Acquisition Considerations

- Breathing and cardiac motion can create significant motion induced artifacts.

  - Breathing motion induced artifacts can be mitigated by breath holding.

    - Typically people can hold their breath for 15–20 s comfortably.

  - Cardiac motion induced artifacts are minimized by ECG gating.

    - The system begins acquiring data after a trigger (typically the QRS complex) and subsequent user defined interval (trigger delay).
    - An acquisition window is set which corresponds to the most quiescent periods of the cardiac cycle (most often diastole).

      - The wider the acquisition window, the more time there is to acquire data (and thus shortens the total time for the scan) but the more susceptible you are to artifact.

    - Regular RR intervals are best for data acquisition and MR systems have arrhythmia rejection algorithms to reduced arrhythmia related artifact.

      - Imaging with irregular heart rates is possible.

    - Both prospective and retrospective gating is possible.

- Averaging acquisitions is a strategy to minimize respiratory motion and to improve SNR but prolongs acquisition time.
- Parallel imaging is a technique that shortens acquisition times by taking advantage of the spatial distribution of the receiving coil (usually a coil array). Essentially, the data is "under-sampled" and the missing data is subsequently reconstructed, "filling in" the gaps.

- Recent advances have allowed free breathing acquisitions by using a "navigator" that tracks the motion of the diaphragm and only acquires data at the same part of the respiratory cycle.

  - Eliminates breath holding, but lengthens scan time as images are only acquired when portion of the respiratory cycle is aligned with cardiac cycle.

Basic CMR Techniques

- Spin Echo Imaging

  - Uses slice selective 90° pulse followed by 180° refocusing pulse.

    - If blood flow is rapid enough for all the blood receiving the first pulse to flow out of the slice, then a signal void is created and images have a "black blood" appearance (Fig. 19.1).
    - Slow moving structures (myocardium, blood vessel walls etc.) appear bright.
    - Provides high contrast between blood and tissue and as such is good for anatomical imaging.
    - Good for both T1 and T2 weighted images.

Tissue characterization

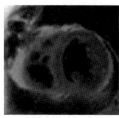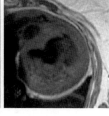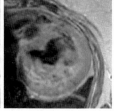

FIGURE 19.1 Tissue Characterization. Short axis T2 weighted (*left*) transverse T1 pregadolinium (*middle*) and transverse T1 post gadolinium (*right*) black blood MR images of the heart. These sequences are for tissue characterization to assess for myocardial edema, fatty metaplasia, infiltration and inflammation

- Areas of high water content (edema, acute injury) in T2 weighted images appear bright.
- Relatively insensitive to magnetic susceptibility artifacts (T2* effects).
- Relatively long TR is required which limits image acquisition speed.
- Slow blood flow can result in more blood signal (brighter) and poor contrast.

    - Inconsistent black blood effect can be overcome with black blood preparation schemes (e.g. dual inversion recovery preparation pulse).

- Gradient Echo Imaging

  - Uses a single rf pulse (flip angle usually between 0 and 90°) to generate the signal.

    - Inflowing blood is fully magnetized and therefore appears bright ("bright blood" imaging).
    - Myocardium and other structures appear grey (intermediate signal intensity) compared to blood.
    - Very short TR allows for high temporal resolution making it good for functional imaging.

        - Used to create cine images to assess cardiac wall motion and function.

    - Relatively sensitive to magnetic susceptibility artifacts (T2* effects).

        - Sternal wires and metallic valves can cause artifacts.
        - Effect can be exploited to assess iron overload in the heart in hemochromatosis.

    - Turbulent blood flow can cause dephasing and thus give a qualitative estimate of stenotic or regurgitant lesions

  - Balanced Steady State Free Precession (bSSFP)

    - Also called FIESTA (GE), TrueFISP (Siemens), or b-FFE (Philips).

- Uses a low flip angle, gradient echo pulse sequence.
- Signal achieves a steady state.
- Has both T1 and T2 weighting (hence "balanced").
- High contrast between blood and myocardium.
- Most commonly used sequence for cardiac function but also good enough resolution to provide structural detail.

- Phase Contrast (PC) Imaging

  - Also called velocity encoding.
  - Can manipulate the MR signal to quantify shifts in the phase of moving spins within a magnetic field yielding information on velocity and direction of movement of the spins.
  - Can quantify (ml/min) blood flow through an orifice (regurgitant or stenotic) which is useful for

    - Valve lesions.
    - Shunt size and shunt fractions (Qp/Qs).
    - Vascular stenosis (coarctation, pulmonary artery stenosis, bypass grafts).

  - Magnitude of phase shift that is measured is angle dependent and so slice selection is paramount.

- Perfusion Imaging

  - Myocardial perfusion studies are usually based on imaging the transit of Gd based contrast through cardiac chambers and then through the myocardial perfusion bed.

    - Most sequences are T1-weighted gradient echo sequences covering multiple slices of the heart at a high temporal resolution.
    - Also called "first pass" perfusion.

- Late Gadolinium Enhancement (LGE)

  - Image myocardium 10–20 min after administration of Gd using an inversion recovery sequence.
  - Gd redistributes into the interstitial spaces before renal clearance.

- Disease processes that increase extracellular volume (focal infiltrative diseases, fibrosis and scar) will result in increased accumulation of Gd that can be imaged and quantified.
- Can assess acute injury patterns (acute MI, myocarditis) as well as chronic injury patterns (chronic infarct, fibrosis).
- Transmural extent of infarction is prognostic and predicts functional improvement after revascularization.
- The pattern of LGE can help determine the etiology of a cardiomyopathy (Table 19.2).

- MR Angiography Imaging

  - Useful for aorta, carotid arteries, renal arteries and peripheral arteries
  - Can use a combination of dark blood and bright blood techniques to finely resolve anatomic detail.

    - Contrast enhancement with Gd can evaluate blood flow through vessel lumens and complex cardiac structures in any orientation allowing for 3-D reconstruction of vascular trees.

Applications for CMR

- Myocardial Ischemia

  - Perfusion scans using Gd and T1 weighted imaging can identify resting perfusion deficits ("first pass" perfusion).
  - Scans can be repeated under stress conditions with vasodilators or dobutamine and is appropriate in people with intermediate pre-test probability of CAD or uninterpretable ECG or unable to exercise.

    - The CE-MARC study (prospective trial of more than 600 patients) found that CMR had a sensitivity of 86 %, specificity of 83 %, positive predictive value of 77 % and negative predictive value of 91 % for detecting myocardial ischemia.

TABLE 19.2 Patterns of LGE

Disease	LGE pattern	LGE location
Myocardial Ischemia	Subendocardial with variable transmural extent	Coronary distribution
Myocarditis	Midwall and Subepicardial	Any location though parvovirus has predilection for lateral wall
Chagas	Midwall and Epicardial	Any location though predilection for inferolateral and apex
Non Ischemic Dilated Cardiomyopathy	Midwall	Any location though predilection for septum
Hypertrophic Cardiomyopathy	Midwall	Patchy often worse at thickest portions of LV. RV insertion sites into LV also common locations.
Arrhythmogenic Right Ventricular Cardiomyopathy	Difficult to determine as RV structure is so thin walled	Any location and can extend the entire length of the RV depending on extent of disease.
Sarcoidosis	Any pattern	Any location including RV
Amyloidosis	Typically diffuse, subendocardial	Any location though can be circumferential
Endomyocardial Fibrosis	Subendocardial	Apex
Anderson-Fabry	Midwall and Epicardial	Inferolateral base

- Significantly better sensitivity and negative predictive values than SPECT.
- Significantly better sensitivity and specificity compared to dobutamine stress echo.

- Additional information obtained during ischemia protocols (wall motion, aortic flow, LGE) adds incremental prognostic value and is predictive of adverse outcomes.
- Role of CMR in acute coronary syndromes is unclear but it is indicated for differentiating STEMI from aortic dissection in patients where this distinction is not clearly evident (Class I, Level B).

- Myocardial Viability (Figs. 19.2 and 19.3)

  - Extent of LGE is associated with functional recovery after coronary revascularization

    - Only 10 % of segments with >50 % transmural enhancement showed functional recovery.
    - Segments with 0–25 % transmural LGE had highest likelihood of recovery.

  - Microvascular obstruction, seen as dark areas surrounded by hyperenhancing (LGE) myocardium, suggests regions where Gd cannot penetrate.

    - Prognostic of post-infarct complications and a better predictor of adverse events than total infarct size.

- Non-ischemic Dilated Cardiomyopathy

  - CMR is the gold standard for chamber volumes and function (Fig. 19.4).

    - Following chamber volumes over time (progressive dilation) and presence of LGE (often midwall) is associated with adverse events.

  - CMR particularly useful when prior testing modalities are discordant or technically limited.
  - Large variety of pulse sequences can provide excellent tissue characterization that can diagnose or exclude specific disease processes.

Viable myocardium

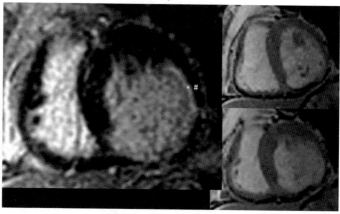

FIGURE 19.2 Viable Myocardium. Late Gadolinium Enhancement in the anterolateral wall of the left ventricle at the basal level (*left image*) involves less than 50 % wall thickness in a subendocardial distribution in the circumflex coronary artery distribution. This segment is likely to recover function following revascularizaton. End diastolic (*top right*) and end systolic (*bottom right image*) white blood images in left ventricular short axis demonstrate hypokinesis in the same segment consistent with hibernating myocardium. On the same images the inferior wall demonstrates nearly transmural late gadoinium enhancement and thinning/akinesis on the white blood cine images, consistent with nonviable myocardium in the posterior descending coronary artery distribution. Late gadolinium enhancement (*), normal myocardium (#)

- Hypertrophic Cardiomyopathy
    - Frequent referral to CMR for evaluation of LVH seen by echo and to exclude HCM.
    - CMR particularly useful in evaluating all myocardial segments.
        - Not constrained by body habitus or viewing windows.
        - Useful in identifying variant patterns of HCM (apical, lateral wall)

Non-viable

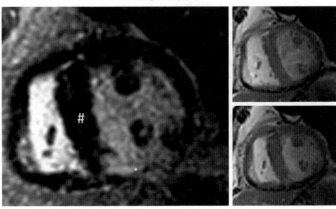

FIGURE 19.3 Nonviable Myocardium. Late Gadolinium Enhancement in the inferior wall of the left ventricle at the mid level (*left image*) is transmural, indication that functional recovery with revascularization is very unlikely. End diastolic (*top right*) and end systolic (*bottom right image*) white blood images in left ventricular short axis demonstrate akinesis in the inferior wall, matching the area of late gadolinium enhancement, consistent with old infarction and scarring. Late gadolinium enhancement (*), normal myocardium (#)

LV volume tracings-method of discs

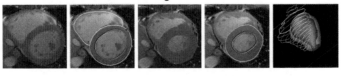

FIGURE 19.4 LV volume tracings. LV cavity in short axis planes are traced to measure LV volumes by method of discs (Simpson's) and calculate LV ejection fraction

- Quantification of LV myocardial mass.
- Able to visualize systolic anterior motion of the mitral valve leaflet and quantify obstruction using phase contrast imaging.
- Can quantify degree of mitral regurgitation.
- LGE tends to be patchy and mid-wall.

- Most commonly at thickest portions of the LV and at RV insertion sites on the septum.
- Any amount of LGE is associated with worse prognosis.

- Arrhythmogenic Right Ventricular Cardiomyopathy

  - Frequent referral for CMR because of unique ability of CMR to evaluate the RV in great detail.
  - Rare disease.
  - Diagnosis cannot be made on imaging criteria alone.
  - CMR exam should focus on quantification of RV volume, function and morphology specifically looking for focal aneurysms and areas of focal RV dysfunction.
  - Although part of the disease pathology, fatty infiltration and fibrosis are not part of the most recent Task Force (2010) criteria as they may be less specific to the disease.

- Non-Compaction Cardiomyopathy

  - CMR is able to define hypertrabeculated myocardium as well as regional dilation and wall motion abnormalities associated with the disease.
  - CMR is able to visualize LV thrombus.
  - A ratio of non-compacted to compacted myocardium of greater than 2.3 (at end diastole) is 86 % sensitive and 99 % specific for diagnosis.

    - However a more recent study using the MESA cohort found that a ratio of >2.3 in at least one myocardial segment was seen in 43 % of normal people.
    - Further validation of CMR parameters for LV non-compaction is necessary to determine optimal diagnostic thresholds.

- Myocarditis

  - Using T2, T1 and Gd contrast enhanced imaging, CMR is able to evaluate edema, hyperemia, necrosis and scar formation.

- CMR is the only non-invasive imaging tool to detect myocardial injury.
- Myocardial T2 and T1 signal is compared to skeletal muscle to assess if there is a relative signal increase in the heart to suggest inflammation.

– Myocardial function and presence of effusions can add additional diagnostic information.

- CMR can also assess pericardial involvement.

– The presence of 2 of 3 CMR criteria (LGE, increased T2 signal, increased early global relative Gd enhancement (T1 signal)) for myocarditis has a sensitivity of 67 % and specificity of 91 %.
– Presence of LGE predicts a worse prognosis and course of disease.

- LGE pattern is typically epicardial or mid-myocardial.

- Sarcoidosis

  – T2 and T1 imaging with Gd (early enhancement) can detect acute inflammation.
  – Assessment of structure and function (wall motion abnormalities at sites of infiltration) can add diagnostic information.
  – Scout images can show mediastinal and hilar adenopathy.
  – LGE imaging can detect areas of focal scar and fibrosis

    - Can be in any distribution (Table 19.2)
    - Amount of LGE is predictive of future adverse events.

  – Can use CMR to follow treatment course and CMR findings often used to help with the decision to place an ICD.

- Amyloidosis

  – CMR can detect cardiac amyloidosis with high sensitivity (88 %) and specificity (90 %).

- Significant accumulation of Gd in the extracellular space that results in Gd being cleared from the blood quickly.
- If fibrosis is extensive you may not see focal areas of LGE as the Gd is evenly distributed.

  - If amyloidosis is suspected, performing LGE imaging earlier (3–5 min post injection) may reveal a typical global subendocardial LGE pattern in LV and RV.
  - LGE of atrial walls may also be present.

- Structural and functional imaging may reveal typical biventricular hypertrophy with biatrial enlargement.

- Cardiac Iron Overload
  - CMR can quantify LV and RV size and function.
  - T2* measurements on gradient echo imaging can be used to identify patients with iron overload in the heart (hereditary hemochromatosis, thalassemia with transfusion dependency, etc.)

    - T2* values <20 ms have been associated with increased likelihood of heart failure and adverse cardiac events.

  - Can use cardiac T2* to monitor chelation therapy.

    - More effective than serial liver biopsies.

- Valvular Heart Disease
  - CMR is valuable for stenotic and regurgitant lesions.
  - Multiple methods for assessing degree of valvular dysfunction.

    - Qualitative assessments can be made using cine gradient echo sequences or bSSFP (Fig. 19.5).

      - Can visualize dephasing caused by turbulent blood flow.
      - Choice of TE can alter this effect and so qualitative assessment of valvular disease needs to be interpreted cautiously.

Dephasing jet

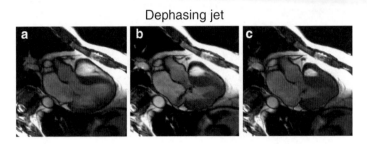

Figure 19.5 Valvular regurgitation detected by dephasing jet. 3 chamber images from white blood SSFP sequence demonstrate early (**a**), mid (**b**) and late (**c**) systole. In mid systole when there is a large pressure gradient between the left ventricle and left atrium a posteriorly directed mitral regurgitation jet (*blue*) arrow is seen as funnel-shaped loss of signal extending into the left atrium from the mitral orifice

- Quantitative assessments can be made using planimetry or using phase contrast imaging (described above).
    - Can determine peak velocity across a valve as well as regurgitant volumes.
    - Can also determine regurgitant volume by taking the difference between RV and LV volume measurements (assumes only a single valvular lesion is present)
  - Importantly, CMR accurately quantifies the degree of dysfunction (i.e. EF or chamber size) resulting from valvular disease.
  - Cine gradient echo images can occasionally visualize vegetations that may be causing valvular regurgitation but that depends on size and location of vegetation
    - However, if a large relatively non-mobile vegetation or mass is seen, the tissue contrast options that CMR can uniquely provide (T1, T2, T2*, fat saturation) allows for the mass to be well characterized.
- Cardiac Masses
  - CMR offers unique tool-kit to assess cardiac masses.

LV apical thrombus

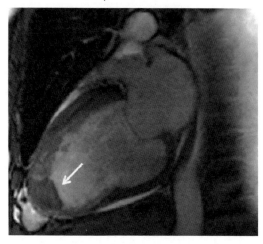

FIGURE 19.6 Excellent spatial resolution allows detection of LV apical thrombus (*arrow*)

- Can differentiate intracavitary thrombus (very sensitive) (Fig. 19.6), benign and malignant lesions.
- The strengths of CMR for this purpose include:
  - Multiplanar image acquisition with high spatial resolution that is independent of body habitus and windowing.
  - Tissue contrast options allow for excellent characterization of the mass including fat content and thrombus association.
  - First pass perfusion imaging can assess the vascularity of the mass.
  - Large field of view allows for visualizing potentially complimentary findings (pleural effusions, mediastinal lymph nodes etc.).

- Congenital Heart Disease
  - CMR is excellent for visualizing anomalous anatomy (3D bSSFP sequences particularly good for this),

quantifying shunt flow (Qp:Qs) and quantifying the sequelae of congenital heart disease (LV and RV mass, volume and ejection fraction).

- Ability to acquire images in any tomographic plane is ideal for assessing congenital lesions that may take unpredictable or tortuous courses.
- Useful in pediatric cases so as to avoid ionizing radiation and follow lesions over time in order to pick the optimal time for intervention.
- Useful in post-intervention setting to follow blood flow through conduits and surgically altered structures (e.g. post Mustard or Jatene, post Fontan, post tetralogy of Fallot repair).
- PC imaging allows you to quantify collateral blood flow across vascular stenosis as well as quantify the contribution of individual vascular structures to overall blood flow (e.g. contribution of each vena cava to pulmonary blood flow post Fontan, assessing anomalous pulmonary and systemic venous return).
- LGE in repaired Tetralogy of Fallot may be predictive of adverse outcomes.

• Pericardial Disease

- CMR is useful to help distinguish between constrictive and restrictive disease.
- CMR allows you to visualize pericardial anatomy (thickening, masses, etc.) and functional consequences of abnormal pericardium.
- CMR features consistent with pericardial constriction include:

  • Pericardial thickness ≥ 4 mm (with or without calcification).
  • Morphologic sequelae such as flattened interventricular septum and dilated hepatic veins.
  • Real time free breathing cine CMR can demonstrate ventricular interdependence.
  • "Septal Bounce" can be visualized with cine imaging.

Tagging for pericardial assessment

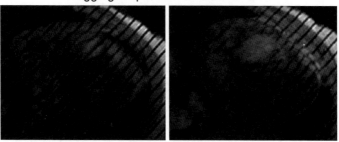

FIGURE 19.7 Tagging for pericardial assessment. Tagging lines across the pericardium should break as the visceral pericardium slides passed the parietal pericardium. Failure of tagging lines to break suggests pericardial adhesions

- Tagged cine imaging can demonstrate areas of regional adhesion (Fig. 19.7)
  - Tagging lines across the pericardium should break as the visceral pericardium slides passed the parietal pericardium.
    - Failure of tagging lines to break suggests pericardial adhesions.

- Pulmonary Vein and Left Atrial Anatomy
  - CMR with contrast can be used to map pulmonary veins and left atrial anatomy prior to radio frequency ablation (RFA).
  - Comparison of pulmonary vein ostial size pre and post ablation can indicate pulmonary vein stenosis, a complication of RFA.

Selected Bibliography

1. Lee VS. Cardiovascular MR, imaging: physical principles to practical protocols. Philadelphia: Lippincott Williams & Wilkins; 2005.
2. Levine GN, Gomes AS, Arai AE, et al. Safety of magnetic resonance imaging in patients with cardiovascular devices: an

American Heart Association scientific statement from the Committee on Diagnostic and Interventional Cardiac Catheterization, Council on Clinical Cardiology, and the Council on Cardiovascular Radiology and Intervention: endorsed by the American College of Cardiology Foundation, the North American Society for Cardiac Imaging, and the Society for Cardiovascular Magnetic Resonance. Circulation. 2007;116:2878–91.

3. Hendel RC, Patel MR, Kramer CM, et al. ACCF/ACR/SCCT/SCMR/ASNC/NASCI/SCAI/SIR 2006 appropriateness criteria for cardiac computed tomography and cardiac magnetic resonance imaging: a report of the American College of Cardiology Foundation Quality Strategic Directions Committee Appropriateness Criteria Working Group, American College of Radiology, Society of Cardiovascular Computed Tomography, Society for Cardiovascular Magnetic Resonance, American Society of Nuclear Cardiology, North American Society for Cardiac Imaging, Society for Cardiovascular Angiography and Interventions, and Society of Interventional Radiology. J Am Coll Cardiol. 2006;48:1475–97.

4. Hundley WG, Bluemke DA, Finn JP, et al. ACCF/ACR/AHA/NASCI/SCMR 2010 expert consensus document on cardiovascular magnetic resonance: a report of the American College of Cardiology Foundation Task Force on Expert Consensus Documents. J Am Coll Cardiol. 2010;55:2614–62.

5. Kim RJ, Fieno DS, Parrish TB, et al. Relationship of MRI delayed contrast enhancement to irreversible injury, infarct age, and contractile function. Circulation. 1999;100:1992–2002.

6. Kim RJ, Wu E, Rafael A, et al. The use of contrast-enhanced magnetic resonance imaging to identify reversible myocardial dysfunction. N Engl J Med. 2000;343:1445–53.

7. Friedrich MG, Sechtem U, Schulz-Menger J, et al. Cardiovascular magnetic resonance in myocarditis: a JACC white paper. J Am Coll Cardiol. 2009;53:1475–87.

8. Mahrholdt H, Wagner A, Deluigi CC, et al. Presentation, patterns of myocardial damage, and clinical course of viral myocarditis. Circulation. 2006;114:1581–90.

9. Patel MR, Cawley PJ, Heitner JF, et al. Detection of myocardial damage in patients with sarcoidosis. Circulation. 2009;120:1969–77.

10. Maceira AM. Cardiovascular magnetic resonance in cardiac amyloidosis. Circulation. 2005;111:186–93.

11. Falk RH. Cardiac amyloidosis: a treatable disease, often overlooked. Circulation. 2011;124:1079–85.

12. Kramer CM, Barkhausen J, Flamm SD, Kim RJ, Nagel E, Society for Cardiovascular Magnetic Resonance Board of Trustees Task Force on Standardized Protocols. Standardized cardiovascular magnetic resonance (CMR) protocols 2013 update. J Cardiovasc Magn Reson. 2013;15:91.

13. Greenwood JP, Maredia N, Younger JF, et al. Cardiovascular magnetic resonance and single-photon emission computed tomography for diagnosis of coronary heart disease (CE-MARC): a prospective trial. Lancet. 2012;379:453–60.

14. Moon JCC, McKenna WJ, McCrohon JA, Elliott PM, Smith GC, Pennell DJ. Toward clinical risk assessment in hypertrophic cardiomyopathy with gadolinium cardiovascular magnetic resonance. J Am Coll Cardiol. 2003;41:1561–7.

15. Olivotto I, Maron BJ, Appelbaum E, et al. Spectrum and clinical significance of systolic function and myocardial fibrosis assessed by cardiovascular magnetic resonance in hypertrophic cardiomyopathy. Am J Cardiol. 2010;106:261–7.

16. Marcus FI, McKenna WJ, Sherrill D, et al. Diagnosis of arrhythmogenic right ventricular cardiomyopathy/dysplasia: proposed modification of the task force criteria. Circulation. 2010;121:1533–41.

17. Petersen SE, Selvanayagam JB, Wiesmann F, et al. Left ventricular non-compaction: insights from cardiovascular magnetic resonance imaging. J Am Coll Cardiol. 2005;46:101–5.

18. Kawel N, Nacif M, Arai AE, et al. Trabeculated (noncompacted) and compact myocardium in adults: the multi-ethnic study of atherosclerosis. Circ Cardiovasc Imaging. 2012;5:357–66.

19. Anderson LJ, Holden S, Davis B, et al. Cardiovascular T2-star (T2*) magnetic resonance for the early diagnosis of myocardial iron overload. Eur Heart J. 2001;22:2171–9.

20. John AS, Dill T, Brandt RR, et al. Magnetic resonance to assess the aortic valve area in aortic stenosis. J Am Coll Cardiol. 2003;42:519–26.

21. Djavidani B, Debl K, Lenhart M, et al. Planimetry of mitral valve stenosis by magnetic resonance imaging. J Am Coll Cardiol. 2005;45:2048–53.

22. O'Donnell DH, Abbara S, Chaithiraphan V, et al. Cardiac tumors: optimal cardiac MR sequences and spectrum of imaging appearances. Am J Roentgenol. 2009;193:377–87.

23. Lotz J, Meier C, Leppert A, Galanski M. Cardiovascular flow measurement with phase-contrast MR imaging: basic facts and implementation. Radiographics. 2002;22:651–71.

24. Axel L. Assessment of pericardial disease by magnetic resonance and computed tomography. J Magn Reson Imaging. 2004;19:816–26.
25. Bogaert J, Francone M. Cardiovascular magnetic resonance in pericardial diseases. J Cardiovasc Magn Reson. 2009;11:14.
26. Axel L, Montillo A, Kim D. Tagged magnetic resonance imaging of the heart: a survey. Med Image Anal. 2005;9:376–93.

Chapter 20
Positron Emission Tomography

Parmanand Singh

PET-Derived MBF and CFR

- Offers a thorough assessment of vascular disease burden by yielding incremental data to SPECT on the presence of disease within the coronary microcirculation.
- For example, in symptomatic patients with established or suspected CAD, SPECT MPI is accurate for identifying flow-limiting or obstructive epicardial coronary disease [1].
- In contrast to SPECT, in multi-vessel epicardial CAD, PET-derived myocardial blood flow (MBF) and coronary flow reserve (CFR) not subjected to balanced ischemia, thereby abrogating the risk of underestimating disease severity [2, 3].
- In addition, early stages of subclinical CAD, which result in microvascular dysfunction may go undetected with standard SPECT MPI [4].
- The additive data on coronary microvascular integrity with PET refines risk stratification in patients with early stages of CAD.

P. Singh, MD
Division of Cardiology, Department of Radiology,
Weill Cornell Medical College, New York Presbyterian Hospital,
New York, NY, USA
e-mail: pas9062@med.cornell.edu

D. Kireyev, J. Hung (eds.), *Cardiac Imaging in Clinical Practice*, In Clinical Practice,
DOI 10.1007/978-3-319-21458-0_20,
© Springer International Publishing Switzerland 2016

- Abnormal MBF and CFR values influence therapeutic management [5].
- In addition, in patients without epicardial CAD, impaired hyperemic CFR and MBF independently predicts development of CAD and increased risk of CV mortality [6, 7].
- Since CAD related functional abnormalities of the coronary artery microcirculation precede anatomical manifestations [5, 8], PET MPI is uniquely positioned to identify at risk individuals, a group that is under diagnosed and may benefit from earlier intervention.

Viability Assessment by PET

- Assessment of myocardial viability with FDG PET in chronic myocardial dysfunction underlying ischemic cardiomyopathy is based on its ability to distinguish between the two pathogenic mechanisms: (i) irreversible loss of myocardium to myocardial infarction (fibrosis/scar) and (ii) at least partially reversible loss of contractility as a result of chronic ischemia (i.e. hibernating myocardium).
- Revascularization has the potential to restore contractile function of hibernating myocardium but not fibrosis/scar [9].
- FDG-PET myocardial viability assessment integrates rest perfusion with myocardial glucose metabolism imaging.
- PET myocardial perfusion imaging (MPI) is superior to SPECT due to improved sensitivity, diagnostic accuracy and lower radiation exposure [10].
- For FDG imaging, patients are studied after an oral glucose load. If the patient has glucose intolerance or diabetes, supplemental insulin will be required.
- Comparison of perfusion and metabolism images can yield one of four common patterns (Table 20.1).

TABLE 20.1 Classification system for flow-metabolism patterns in FDG-PET myocardial viability studies

Perfusion	Glucose metabolism	Category
Preserved	Preserved	Viable
Reduced	Preserved	Mismatch (viable hibernation)
Reduced	Reduced	Match (non-viable)
Preserved	Reduced	Reverse mismatch (altered regional glucose metabolism)

References

1. Shaw LJ, Min JK, Hachamovitch R, et al. Cardiovascular imaging research at the crossroads. JACC Cardiovasc Imaging. 2010;3:316–24.
2. Mc Ardle BA, Dowsley TF, de Kemp RA, Wells GA, Beanlands RS. Does rubidium-82 PET have superior accuracy to SPECT perfusion imaging for the diagnosis of obstructive coronary disease?: a systematic review and meta-analysis. J Am Coll Cardiol. 2012;60:1828–37.
3. Ziadi MC, Dekemp RA, Williams K, et al. Does quantification of myocardial flow reserve using rubidium-82 positron emission tomography facilitate detection of multivessel coronary artery disease? J Nucl Cardiol. 2012;19:670–80.
4. Schwaiger M, Muzik O. Assessment of myocardial perfusion by positron emission tomography. Am J Cardiol. 1991;67:35D–43.
5. Camici PG, Crea F. Coronary microvascular dysfunction. N Engl J Med. 2007;356:830–40.
6. Herzog BA, Husmann L, Valenta I, et al. Long-term prognostic value of 13N-ammonia myocardial perfusion positron emission tomography added value of coronary flow reserve. J Am Coll Cardiol. 2009;54:150–6.
7. Murthy VL, Naya M, Foster CR, et al. Association between coronary vascular dysfunction and cardiac mortality in patients with and without diabetes mellitus. Circulation. 2012;126:1858–68.
8. Bengel FM, Higuchi T, Javadi MS, Lautamaki R. Cardiac positron emission tomography. J Am Coll Cardiol. 2009;54:1–15.

9. Marwick TH, MacIntyre WJ, Lafont A, Nemec JJ, Salcedo EE. Metabolic responses of hibernating and infarcted myocardium to revascularization. A follow-up study of regional perfusion, function, and metabolism. Circulation. 1992;85:1347–53.

10. Slart RH, Bax JJ, van Veldhuisen DJ, et al. Prediction of functional recovery after revascularization in patients with chronic ischaemic left ventricular dysfunction: head-to-head comparison between 99mTc-sestamibi/18F-FDG DISA SPECT and 13N-ammonia/18F-FDG PET. Eur J Nucl Med Mol Imaging. 2006;33:716–23.

Index

D. Kireyev, J. Hung (eds.), *Cardiac Imaging in Clinical Practice*, In Clinical Practice,
DOI 10.1007/978-3-319-21458-0,
© Springer International Publishing Switzerland 2016

Made in the USA
Lexington, KY
09 February 2017